Ab

Tony Sheldon was born on 19 November 1953, which makes him a Scorpio. He is told by people who know about such things that this is nothing to be proud of.

He attended Bellevue Hill Public School and became school captain, which meant he had to lead the school pledge at assembly on Monday mornings.

From there he went to Sydney Boys High School, rode surfboards and bleached his hair to attract girls.

At the end of high school he had to decide what he wanted to do with the rest of his life.

At first he thought he might study medicine, as he'd always done well at school, and it seemed to him that if a person was smart and Jewish there was some unwritten obligation to become a doctor. Unfortunately for Tony, being around sick people made him nauseous. Being a vet seemed like a reasonable alternative.

He has run his own inner-city practices for fifteen years. Prior to that he worked in half a dozen other practices in Australia and overseas.

TO DAD,
WHO SHOULD HAVE
BEEN HERE TO SHARE THIS

The trouble with HARVEY

Tales of a city vet

TONY SHELDON

HarperCollinsPublishers

Harper*Collins**Publishers***

First published in Australia in 1997
by HarperCollins*Publishers* Pty Limited
ACN 009 913 517
A member of the HarperCollins*Publishers* (Australia) Pty Limited Group

HarperCollins*Publishers*
25 Ryde Road, Pymble, Sydney NSW 2073, Australia
31 View Road, Glenfield, Auckland 10, New Zealand
77–85 Fulham Palace Road, London W6 8JB, United Kingdom
Hazelton Lanes, 55 Avenue Road, Suite 2900, Toronto, Ontario M5R 3L2
and 1995 Markham Road, Scarborough, Ontario M1B 5M8, Canada
10 East 53rd Street, New York NY 10032, USA

National Library of Australia Cataloguing-in-Publication data:

Sheldon, Tony, 1953– .
The trouble with Harvey : tales of a city vet.
ISBN 0 7322 5764 6.
1. Pets – Anecdotes. 2. Veterinary medicine – Anecdotes.
I. Title.
A828.302

Cover photograph by Louise Lister
Printed in Australia by McPherson's Printing Group

9 8 7 6 5 4 3 2 1
99 98 97

Contents

1 Super stud 7

2 In the beginning 13

3 The last supper 29

4 Cuddle Pie 43

5 The trouble with Harvey 50

6 The pyramid 61

7 Skin deep 68

8 Bedside manner 76

9 Tactical response 88

10 Rainy days and Mondays 97

11 Fat chance 105

12 Old troupers 113

13 Glasnost in Surry Hills 123

14 Love is blind 133

15 Death wish 139

16 Performance art 153

17 On another plane 168

18 Blind faith 184

19 Over the fence 194

20 Dotty about Dottie 203

21 Captured on camera 213

chapter 1

Super Stud

Norbert was the most magnificent Great Dane. Ninety-four centimetres to the shoulder, tan all over, with a moderate blackening of the muzzle. A quiet brooding strength. During periods of mayhem in the waiting room Norbert would just stand there like the Colossus of Rhodes, disdainfully watching the idiocy of his surroundings.

Norbert's breeding was impeccable. His ancestry was strewn with Grand Champions and Best of Breed, and he walked like he knew it, with a regal loping stride and his head held high. He was quite a contrast to Miss Grimshaw, who had poorly dyed, shoulder-length, stringy red hair, and was one of those roundish people who always seem to have a sunburnt face. And, at around 155 centimetres tall and weighing about eighty kilos, she had an unfortunate penchant for wearing body-hugging tracksuits and jogging shoes. Miss Grimshaw would always sit in the waiting room with her hands in her lap, his majesty proudly by her side.

It's the most wonderful trait of dogs — their unconditional love and loyalty unswayed by wealth, beauty and dress sense, all of which Miss Grimshaw was somewhat lacking.

Norbert appeared to have one weakness, however — his fertility. Because he was such a stunner at all the dog shows, Miss Grimshaw was inundated with requests for his services as a stud. Unfortunately his success rate at getting his partners pregnant was abysmal and so here he was, being admitted to the hospital for a sperm count.

Our nurse at this time was a lovely, shy, conscientious sixteen-year-old girl by the name of Felicity, who, sadly, was burdened with a fairly severe stutter. She was in the waiting room when Miss Grimshaw and Norbert arrived.

"Hi, Miss Grimshaw. N . . . N . . . Norbert's looking well, isn't he," Felicity said, stating the obvious. "What's he here for?"

"Sperm count."

"Oh! Oh! I'll t . . . t . . . tell T . . . T . . . Tony. I'm sure he w . . . w . . . won't be t . . . t . . . too long." When compromised, Felicity's stutter would deteriorate appreciably.

A few minutes later I motioned Miss Grimshaw and Norbert into the surgery. "Felicity tells me that you've brought Norbert in for a sperm count."

"That's right, Mr Sheldon," she began confidentially, in a semi whisper. "He doesn't seem to be getting many of the bitches pregnant, you see."

I suggested we keep Norbert in for the day to collect the sample, and that he'd be all right to go home that evening. The sample would be sent to the university for evaluation.

I was then confronted with the task of explaining to Felicity — young, innocent, stuttering Felicity — how we were to approach the procedure.

"Do we have to c . . . c . . . catheterise him?" she asked.

"No, Felicity, not quite." I was unsure how best to approach this delicate issue.

"Then how do we get the sample?"

"We have to masturbate him." I didn't know an easier way of saying it and, what the hell, I knew what that meant when I was sixteen.

Felicity turned crimson. "What do you w . . . w . . . want me to d . . . d . . . do?"

There was this mischievous side of me that wanted to give her the job of manually stimulating Norbert. Fortunately, the good-guy side of me won. I instructed her to take a sterile jar from the cupboard and, when Norbert's joy was brought to fruition, she was to catch it in the jar.

I don't think the idea appealed to Felicity, whose face had now turned from crimson to white. Sweat suddenly appeared on her brow.

"Now, Felicity," I said, "you'll have to be quick and

accurate. The sample's no good once it hits the floor."

She silently walked out into the kennel area and returned with Norbert, his head erect, hers bowed. I explained the technique we were to use and proceeded to get the show on the road.

So there we were, Norbert standing upright, albeit a little glazed of eye as his dignity slowly left him, with me kneeling next to him doing what apparently sends men blind, and Felicity kneeling in front of him, head under his chest, arms outstretched and hands clasped firmly around the jar, waiting for Vesuvius to erupt. She was wide eyed and focused. That mischievous side of me was having an unacceptably good time. I'm sure Felicity felt that this wasn't part of her job description.

Twenty minutes later nothing had happened. I was sure my technique was good, so perhaps it was the environment that wasn't conducive to total fulfilment.

At the time I was living in the flat above the hospital, and so I suggested to Felicity that we take Norbert upstairs to continue the procedure. Maybe playing some romantic music on my stereo would put him more in the mood.

"OK," she said quietly. "If you th . . . think that would help."

So we took the phones off the hook, headed upstairs and played a Charles Aznavour record. We lay Norbert on his side this time and began the process all over again. The music may well have relaxed him. It didn't relax Felicity — hands again clasped tightly around the jar, arms outstretched, eyes wide and focused.

Still nothing happened. We could get him erect, but that's as far as it went. We persevered for another fifteen to twenty minutes, but I was getting a cramp in my hand and Felicity was visibly tiring.

"This isn't working," I begrudgingly admitted.

Then a flash of genius. Boarding at our other hospital was a Beagle on heat. Her owners had left her with us because they couldn't cope with the mess and the hordes of dogs waiting outside the house. If we were to stand her in front of Norbert we couldn't possibly fail. So I rushed downstairs and across to the other hospital to fetch her.

This short interlude gave Felicity and me a well-earned break. Norbert, too, seemed a little jaded.

I walked in the back door with my temptress and as soon as Norbert saw her I knew the battle was as good as won. His poise was absolutely shattered. This, of course, was going to make Felicity's and my task even harder. She was going to have to hold the Beagle in one hand and the jar in the other, while I stimulated Norbert and tried to hold him back. I didn't want to have to explain Beagle–Great Dane pups to people who had entrusted me with the task of specifically avoiding such an event.

As I had predicted, this time it didn't take long at all. Norbert was spectacular. So was Felicity. Desperately holding the Beagle and trying not to lose any of Norbert's offering, she moved with lightning speed, demonstrating incredible hand–eye co-ordination. This shy girl . . . I never would have thought it. She managed, somehow, to catch about half of it in the jar, the rest landing on various parts of her uniform.

The ordeal now over, Felicity broke into the most wonderful and now not-so-innocent smile. "You enjoyed that, didn't you, Tony?" she said.

Not a hint of a stutter.

chapter 2

In the beginning

Looking back on my days at university I now realise how free of worries they really were. Sure we had exams, but I'd always been good at those, since I had the fortunate ability to remember things easily, which enabled me to get through with a minimum of "hard slog" study. I didn't do brilliantly but I never failed a subject or had to be brought back to do an exam again. Throughout my studies I seemed to do best at the practical stuff, the hands-on work with the animals.

The first three years were pretty boring, especially the first, being bogged down in theory. Chemistry and physics were like a foreign tongue; I never got a decent hold on either and their relevance always eluded me. How could the concept of something called a "Black Hole" in outer space help me diagnose hepatitis in a Springer Spaniel? How could my knowing that if I mixed extra-strong sulphuric acid with just about anything it would still burn a hole in my desk help me fix a Kelpie's broken leg?

Physiology, during the second year, was a little more interesting — although sending electric shocks through a frog's legs to see how fast they twitched didn't exactly thrill me, especially after first knocking out the frog by slamming its head against the top of the desk in a procedure called "pithing" (after which, the frog was said to be "pithed" — like many of the people who passed through the Vet School over the years).

Anatomy was our first real introduction to domestic animals, even if they were all dead. On our first day we were ushered into the Anatomy Lab, where we were confronted by three long, forbidding black benches on which had been placed the embalmed bodies of some twenty to thirty unsuccessful greyhounds. Greyhounds were used because of their minimal body fat, which allowed for better identification of muscles and tendons.

These dogs were preserved in formalin and initially the smell was overwhelming. Our first entry into that room evoked the full range of expletives and nose holding. Each dog was assigned to two or three students who had to systematically dissect it and identify the various body parts.

Our anatomy lecturer was Dr Calvin, a solidly built, well-dressed English gentleman. He loved his subject passionately, always trying to inject a certain dignity into its presentation. He strove for accuracy in the pronunciation of all the Latin names of the bones and muscles. Nevertheless, despite his passion, to most of us anatomy was, at least initially, just cutting up smelly dead dogs. We hadn't yet grasped the bigger picture. At this early stage all we could see were indistinguishable pieces of meat, each with a name like a dead Roman.

I'd never done anything surgical before, and here I was with a razor-sharp scalpel hovering over a reeking, rock-hard corpse. My first incision was tentative. My hand was shaking. How hard was I supposed to press? How far should I make the cut? What if I cut off the wrong bit? I really don't know why I was so concerned. After all, the dog was dead long before I got to it. What further damage could I possibly do?

In time, however, caution gave way to fearless navigation. We cut with reckless abandon, recognising each of the landmarks as we came to them. The names became more familiar and soon we were all travelling in friendlier waters.

On the day we were to sit for our practical anatomy exam at the end of the year we were led into The Room With The Black Benches. To an outsider it would have looked like The Chamber of Horrors. There was a skull, with some muscles still attached, sitting on the end of one bench, an eye still in one of the sockets. Further along, half a leg, skewered with a steel spike to make it stand upright. On another bench, a heart, thankfully not still pumping. There was a liver, a set of lungs still attached to a windpipe, a penis with its usual complement of testicles, and a whole host of other body parts, all arranged neatly on the black benchtops. We were each assigned a questionnaire and had about three minutes at each specimen before moving on to the next.

I passed comfortably, and the next year I graduated to dissecting horses. Obviously we couldn't have a dead horse for every two students, so we had a couple of horses for the entire class and we each took turns cutting them up. These horses were suspended from the ceiling by two giant steel bolts. After the previous year of anatomy we were now relatively immune to such grisly sights and were soon into our horses with zeal.

So desensitised had I become that I was brazen enough to steal a fetlock, take it home with me and put it in the fridge. Including the hoof it was only about 30 centimetres high and so after some rearranging of shelves it fitted in nicely, standing up.

On the following weekend was my father's birthday party. I uncharacteristically volunteered to greet the guests at the front door. I took my fetlock from the fridge and hid it in the sleeve of my jacket.

The doorbell rang. Opening the door with my left hand, I was able to keep my right behind my back.

"Hello, Tony," Uncle Robert said, extending his hand.

It was the opening I'd been waiting for.

"Hi. How are you?" I said, taking my right hand from behind my back.

Uncle Robert shook the horse's hoof, totally unperturbed. I was a tad disappointed, but not discouraged.

Although I didn't send any of the guests running to the bathroom to be sick, most of them were sufficiently disgusted for me to regard the exercise as a success.

As the years progressed at university what we had learnt in theory was put into practice as we were introduced to clinical cases as they came through the hospital. In our fourth year we were divided into groups. Some were placed in clinical rounds where cases were discussed with the clinicians, some assisted with and watched surgery, some helped with radiology, while others were assigned to anaesthetics. It was only at this point that we really felt actively involved in the profession we had chosen.

Final year was spent exclusively, except for weekends, on the University Farms, at Camden, about an hour and a half's drive from Sydney. We had all our lectures and practical work there. It was essentially fourth year on a farm. All the disciplines we practised on small animals the previous year were duplicated with the large animals.

During the first four years of the course it was also mandatory for students to spend a certain part of their vacation time working with the various different species they had studied, or were still to study in the final year. So I found myself working on a dairy farm in Otorohonga, New Zealand (where I learned that it was best not to have one's face too close to a cow's rear while one is fumbling with her teats and a milking machine); on a sheep station near Wagga Wagga, New South Wales (where I learned that, without a sheepdog, two city boys can't succeed in rounding up two thousand sheep merely by running up and down hills and round and round a paddock); and in a small-animal practice in Aspen, Colorado (where I learned not to use my hands to fend off a friendly Samoyed who had so many porcupine quills in him he looked like a sea urchin with nostrils).

Once the joys of university days were behind me, it was time to take off the training wheels and face the real world.

I had an advantage over most of the other keen but very raw new graduates, or at least I thought I did, as an aunt of mine was friendly with a vet in the outer suburbs of Sydney who was looking for an assistant. I phoned for an appointment and drove the forty-five minutes to his surgery. I was nervous but, as they say, cautiously optimistic. My aunt was sure to have painted a glowing picture.

The first thing that struck me about Dr Rossito was the size of his neck. It was so large, certainly wider than his head, and his head wasn't small. It came down like a pyramid onto his shoulders. He had short, straight, black receding hair combed back, and a dark complexion. His large forehead was always shiny. The whole time I worked with him it was never matt . . . always high gloss. And his hair seemed to sprout all the way down the back of that amazing neck.

"You haven't worked anywhere before have you, Tony?"

That was certainly settling. I explained that, while I only graduated two months ago, I had done a lot of small-animal work at university and worked for a couple of months in an Aspen practice. I didn't want to appear totally useless.

"Well, it doesn't matter. I've had many assistants, some experienced, some not. None have been very good."

Another vote of confidence. Surely they couldn't all have been hopeless. Not every single one. I started to wonder how many "many" was. I wondered why none of them had lasted, and if they'd left of their own accord or had been sacked.

"So," he said, interlocking his fingers in front of him on the desk, "when do you think you can start?"

"Any time."

"Good. We'll see you next Monday morning at 8.00."

Just like that? That was all? That was the end of the interview? No questions about my grades, my practical experience or my interests? No small talk about my future plans? I felt oddly let down by the brevity of it all. Except to tell me that every assistant vet he'd ever hired was hopeless, he'd said practically nothing.

I slept only intermittently that night, both excited and anxious about the first step into my new career.

As things turned out it was to be a steep, short step. It was to become the worst job I'd ever had or was to have in my life. Worse than when I had to carry Gyprock plasterboard sheeting up five flights of stairs for an entire day. Worse than the time I spent standing in a menswear store for hours on end telling people they looked good in ridiculous clothes.

Dr Rossito, or just plain Nino as he preferred me to call him, wasn't the only problem. There was also his head nurse, Freda. She looked as one would expect a Freda to look: big, strong and buxom. She was probably in her mid to late thirties. Her hair was short, blonde and severe, and she wore a perfectly pressed neat blue uniform. She had a definite Nordic appearance about her. I could easily visualise her wearing a metal helmet, long fake plaits, singing opera and breaking glass. "Her" hospital, as she liked to refer to it, was run like a labour camp. She usually managed to have at least one of "her" nurses in tears at some point during each day. The turnover of nurses while I was there was even more rapid than the turnover of vets before me.

Nino owned the houses on either side of the hospital. Freda lived in one with her daughter from a previous marriage, while the other was kept vacant for the assistant vet when he was on call for a weekend. "Vacant" was an accurate description. There was one bed (with no sheets), one chair, a telephone, and a temperamental black and white television . . . oh yes, and in the cutlery drawer was a fork. One lonely, bent fork. No plates, no cups no bowls. Just the fork.

The first inkling I had that Nino's practice was going to be a difficult and perhaps unpleasant place to work was when I was stitching up a cat's leg in the operating theatre. It was a simple procedure and so as I worked I chatted with Dominique, one of the nurses who had actually survived there for more than four months, when Nino called out from his office:

"No talking!"

I looked at Dominique in disbelief. "No talking? Aren't we allowed to talk?"

"Not while we're operating," she whispered.

It was like being back at school. And it wasn't a universal rule either. When Nino operated Freda would come in and gush reams of adulation at his surgical prowess.

"Great work, Nino. You're so clever."

He, of course, would lap it up and further describe to her in detail every step of what he was doing, even minor procedures, thus inviting further effusive praise from his surgical groupie. It was revolting.

Sally, one of the other nurses, gave me a nudge as I walked out to do some of the treatments. "She's sleeping with him, you know."

"He can't be," I said. "He's married."

Sally could have said, "You're kidding — grow up," but just looked at me with a worldly smirk.

Nino and Freda would often have lunch together in her house, while I would continue with any surgery or medical work-ups that needed to be done. Occasionally, I would need to get some advice about a case in hospital and I would knock at her door. She would open it only about three centimetres and peering through the crack would answer abruptly: "Yes, what is it?"

Was I contagious? Did I have the plague? I couldn't understand the secrecy, all the cloak and dagger stuff. I could see Nino having lunch at the kitchen table. It was all above board. Everyone was fully clothed.

"Can I have a word with Nino?" I would ask.

She would leave and Nino would then come to the door, but he wouldn't open it any wider than she had.

"Yes, Tony?" he would say, peering through.

I would then explain the problem, and he would advise me — all through that little slit in the door.

The first time I thought it was just a rude oversight. After it happened four or five times I'd break into a nervous sweat trying to summon the courage to knock. I felt like an intruder. It wasn't as if I was asking all that many questions . . . maybe two or three a week. Two months down the track I felt like levering the damn door open with a crowbar.

Nino, I was soon to learn, also had a ferocious temper. I once made the mistake of querying his costing of one of the cases in hospital. It seemed to me inordinately expensive. He took it so personally. It was almost as if I'd defamed him.

"Nino," I said. "I can't understand how you reached that figure."

Well, what ensued made Hiroshima look like a Boy Scout campfire. I really didn't think I'd insulted his entire ancestral lineage. He began to repetitively clench his jaw and twitch. His face started to turn red and then purple. Droplets of sweat appeared on that shiny forehead. His eyes started to glaze over maniacally. And then the giveaway sign that he was about to totally lose control . . . the veins in his temples began to swell and pulsate. I thought his head was about to explode.

I'd never seen anything like it. I felt the life force drain from my body as I stood paralysed waiting for my impending doom. I prayed to whatever god was available to let the ground swallow me up or failing that at least make my death swift and painless. I wanted to be home in bed curled up under the covers. It was only a matter of time before his pressure valve blew.

"There's a lot of things you won't understand, boy!" he screamed. "Don't you ever question my charges! You don't know anything!"

I'd obviously hit a nerve. Nino's head had definitely swelled thirty per cent, and those veins in his temples were throbbing so hard I could have gauged his heart rate from across the street.

Then he started indiscriminately throwing the syringes and needles he was holding in his hands. Not specifically at me, but I was still ducking for cover. This was fast beginning to look like a place where long-service leave wasn't going to be an issue.

Then he stormed out of the room, slamming the door behind him and almost tearing it off its hinges.

The next day it was as though nothing had happened. He was totally unaffected, cheerful and friendly. Of course, I was scarred for life.

These outbursts were unpredictable. I suppose his juggling an affair and a marriage was leaving him frayed around the edges. They could come at any time and could be measured on the Richter scale. As explosive and terrifying as they were, at least they were short. It was, however, starting to sap my confidence. I was becoming hesitant for fear of triggering one of these earthquakes, and starting to doubt my suitability for this profession.

It was little consolation that these tirades weren't reserved only for me. At times he would erupt with the nurses too. Freda would often join in and back him up, like tag-team wrestling. As one would run out of breath the other would step in and continue the onslaught. She was also pretty good at launching solo raids on the girls. I would stand back and watch shocked as they were systematically stripped of their dignity, these onslaughts often entering unnecessary personal areas. I could see why none of them were going to be eligible for long-service either.

It was interesting that Freda never once screamed at me. Perhaps she felt it was outside her jurisdiction.

I got on well with the nurses, and as we worked or had lunch we'd talk about everyday things like movies or what we did on the weekend.

Sadly my most peaceful times at this practice were when one of the nurses and I had to take the dead animals out to the tip. One was certainly grasping at straws if that was a highlight, but it was so good to be away from the minefield.

That particular means of disposing of people's pets also upset me. There was one outside room at the hospital where all the dead animals were kept. They weren't stored in bags or any other type of container. Just piled up on top of each other. When the room was considered full enough or smelly enough we would throw the bodies into the hospital van, drive out and toss them onto the tip. I suppose when you're dead you're dead, but that was someone's very much loved pet and that memory surely deserved better. I vowed that when I had my own place I would have a more compassionate solution.

One afternoon Nino pulled me aside and offered the most ridiculous advice. "Tony, I really don't think you should talk with the nurses."

"Why?"

"They're of a lower mentality."

I couldn't believe what I was hearing.

"What do you mean 'lower mentality'?" I asked. "Lower than what?"

"You'll understand as you get older, believe me."

Well, some twenty years down the track I'm older and I still don't understand. He and Freda always thought the staff were conspiring against them. The truth, of course, was the staff really only wanted the occasional kind word and a little encouragement.

My time there was becoming unbearable. It got to the point that from the moment I arrived in the morning, I couldn't wait to go home. The closer I got to the surgery the more sombre and morose I became. The continual worry that the slightest indiscretion, and not just by me, could lead to the most volatile onslaught of personal abuse was starting to fray me around the edges. Not only was I getting pimples for the first time in my life, I was becoming a different person. Usually happy and outgoing, I was starting to feel like Peter Lorre.

I think the final straw came that Christmas Eve. I was on call that weekend and staying in the very vacant house next to the surgery. It was about nine o'clock and I was sitting in the only seat in the dimly lit lounge room trying to focus on the double images coming from the television. Christmas Eve was always a big family tradition at home and this was the first one I could remember missing when I was home in Australia. It was sad to be spending it with the bent fork. Then the phone rang.

"Hi, Tony. It's Freda. Nino and I are having some roast lamb. Would you like some?"

I was floored. What was this, an olive branch, a

white flag, a burying of the hatchet? Maybe they weren't so bad after all. Maybe I misjudged them and they really did feel the Christmas spirit. Maybe I just got them on a bad month or two. They could see I was lonely and were offering a compassionate hand.

"Yes, I'd love some. That would be wonderful."

I was just about to say "I'll be over in a minute" when she shot me down.

"Good, I'll bring some over for you."

"Oh, OK. Thanks, that's great."

A few seconds later there was a knock at the door. I opened it and there was Freda holding an old chipped plate with a pile of little cut-up pieces of lamb on it. No vegetables, no potatoes, no rice, no salad. No presentation at all. Just an old plate full of little square pieces of meat. And no cutlery. Why didn't they just leave it on the doorstep for me? I felt like dropping to my knees, wagging my tail and licking her feet with unbridled joy.

I took the plate and sat back down in front of the television. I didn't even bother to use my little mate the bent fork. What was the point? It was the final dehumanising straw. I just sat there crying. The saddest thing was that in their effort at what could have been a wonderful gesture they'd treated me like a dog. They just didn't know any better. I knew then I couldn't stay any longer.

The next work day I gave notice.

I felt like I'd finally emerged from a dark tunnel and into brilliant sunshine when I walked out of that practice for the last time. It was like the Allies had landed and I'd been liberated. I felt terrific. I drove home almost weightless. No more ducking for cover from flying syringes, no more speaking through cracks in doors and no more lonely Christmas Eves.

I ate heartily that night, watched a bit of television, took the dog for a walk with Dad, and happily went to bed early. It was surprising that my parents, who always had the attitude that you had to stick with things to the bitter end, were supportive in my decision to leave. They were almost thrilled when I told them I'd given my notice.

I had no idea what the future held, except that it held something new, and whatever that was it would have to be an improvement on where I'd just been.

chapter 3

The last Supper

After a locum stint in Newcastle, it was again time to look for a permanent job. I heard of a partnership that needed someone to manage two city practices, and I wasted no time in phoning one of the vets for an interview. We arranged to meet at a restaurant for lunch.

I arrived a little early because I was keen to make a good first impression and didn't want to keep him waiting. I also had no idea what he looked like. I should have asked the vet how I was to recognise him but I had been too excited on the phone to think of it. Anyway, I figured he'd be the only man walking in on his own at the time we specified. Of course that was a stupid assumption and two embarrassing "Hello, I'm Tony Sheldon" greetings to the wrong people preceded his arrival.

Tim Darkhome came dressed in a tweed jacket,

moleskin trousers and riding boots. I think he saw himself as a bit of a country squire, and he turned out to be quite a talker.

He spoke of how he made a squillion from a practice he once had in the country, and how the two city practices he and Chris Hoskins had opened would be goldmines. Ted talked about many things over the next hour, but mostly he talked about Ted and how successful and rich he'd been in the past.

My first reaction was to wonder how all that wealth had apparently dissipated.

It really wasn't an interview as such. It seemed more that he just wanted to meet the person who was going to run his two practices, and let that person know how great he was. He told me he hadn't interviewed anyone else about the job and had no intention of doing so. I figured he was either incredibly impressed with me or just lazy. As I'd barely been able to get a word in edgeways during our meeting the latter was probably closer to the truth.

Having finished our lunch of oysters, steak and a few drinks the bill arrived and, lo and behold, Tim couldn't find his wallet. He fumbled deliberately in his trousers and jacket for an unnecessarily long time and then unconvincingly proclaimed: "I can't believe it. I must have left my wallet in the car."

"That's OK. I'll look after it," I smiled, and paid the bill.

"I'll give you the money on Monday," he said.

Of course he never did, and the matter was never broached again.

My job was to run and, it was hoped, build up both the new practices on my own. It would mean that I would have to stagger the consulting hours. I would consult at Pyrmont for an hour and a half in the morning and then rush across to Alexandria ten minutes away and consult for another hour and a half there. Then I would do whatever surgery had been scheduled until the afternoon consulting period at Pyrmont. I would have an hour and a half there and then rush across to Alexandria again and consult there. I was to live in the flat above the Alexandria practice and be on call at night. The consulting hours would also be staggered on the weekends but only in the morning. This system worked well initially, but soon business started to pick up and I was getting run off my feet during the day and, being on call seven nights a week, getting limited sleep.

There were also logistical problems. Pyrmont didn't have an X-ray machine, and so any animals that required X-rays I would have to take in my car across to Alexandria. Some days I found myself rushing backwards and forwards like a demented chook. Furthermore, neither place really had enough cages, so on really busy days there would be dogs tied to the operating tables, and cats kept all day in their baskets.

However, despite these problems, and my consequent dwindling social life, I was really enjoying the work, and was proud of the rapid increase in business I had been able to create. And I was continually amazed and entertained by the ridiculous situations I found myself in.

When you start out in practice, naivety often clouds better judgment and you embark on a course which, in hindsight, should well have been approached more cautiously. In this particular case caution was sidestepped altogether.

Having just taken over the management of the two city practices, I naturally wanted to endear myself to prospective clients. One such client was Marlene Hodgekin, a lady who lived blissfully with some twenty-six cats. I felt that to get well acquainted with such a lady would be beneficial to my fledgling practice.

Naivety rarely goes unpunished.

Marlene Hodgekin was probably in her fifties. She lived with Phillip, a thin angular man some years her junior, who had a very sparse excuse for a beard and moustache, and a ready smile which flaunted his not quite full quota of teeth. I had assumed they were married, but Marlene was quick to point out they weren't and, in fact, hadn't made love for six years, a confidence I could have done without.

One evening Marlene phoned the surgery and invited me over for dinner to celebrate Phillip's birthday. I'd always been of the view that it was unwise to become too friendly with clients, but here was a lady with twenty-six cats! And I was trying to build up the practice . . . so, with some trepidation, I accepted.

At the time I was living with a wonderful lady, Yolanda, and I asked Marlene if we could both come. I didn't want to face the evening alone.

"Of course, that would be fine," Marlene cheerfully replied. "We'd love to meet her."

"What time would you like us to arrive?" I asked.

"At 4.30 would be fine."

It seemed unusually early to me, but I just supposed some people ate earlier than others.

I told Yolanda we'd been invited to a birthday dinner for the husband of one of my clients.

"That sounds great."

"Well, he's not actually her husband. They've sort of lived together for a long time, but they haven't had sex for six years."

"That's important. Anything else you'd like to share with me?"

"She's got several cats."

"How many?"

"Twenty-six," I mumbled as I slunk from the room.

"How many?" she yelled after me.

I pretended not to hear, which in our small flat was impossible. She came after me like a power walker.

"How many?"

"Twenty-six," I said meekly.

"Oh my God. That house is going to reek."

That was probably true, but sacrifices had to be made for the betterment of my career.

We arrived punctually at 4.30 and rang the bell. Marlene answered the door, still in her dressing gown.

"I'm so glad you're here, now I can have a shower."

With that she disappeared. Yolanda and I stood in the hallway and just looked at each other, dumbfounded.

"This is not a good start, Tony."

Phillip then ambled in, smiled, and vaguely said hello. And that's all he said as he ambled straight past us. As it turned out he wasn't much of a talker. He just smiled a lot.

Pretty much left to our own devices we started to look around the house, not so much to pry but more to avoid just standing in one place like two shags on a rock.

Even at this early stage I was beginning to feel that my decision to accept this invitation was probably not a very smart one. First impressions don't often let me down, and as the evening went on, mine were to be firmly reinforced.

Firstly I really should have realised that twenty-six cats don't make for a very "guest-welcoming" odour. Yolanda was spot-on. There were litter trays all over the place, some clean, while others looked like they hadn't been cleaned in days.

It seemed nowhere was off limits. There were six cats sitting in the kitchen, one actually in a frying pan on the stove. I nudged Yolanda and whispered: "I hope she's not going to cook our meal in that one."

She didn't get the joke. The evening was not starting well for her.

When she'd had her shower and changed, Marlene offered us a seat on the tattered couch while she prepared dinner. Phillip turned on the TV. So there we three sat, mindlessly watching the TV. Occasionally Phillip would look toward us and smile, and every so often introduce one of the cats that wandered through to use the litter tray next to the couch. But by and large we sat for what seemed like forever in one of those uncomfortable silences. I looked across at Yolanda and with an apologetic smile shrugged my shoulders.

About 6.30 Marlene emerged from the kitchen. "Dinner's ready. Everyone grab some newspaper to put on your laps."

Newspaper! Yolanda turned and looked at me sharply, wide-eyed, jaws clenched.

We all walked over to a pile of old newspapers in the corner and grabbed some.

"Nice touch," I joked weakly as we sat down and placed a section of the *Sydney Morning Herald* on our laps.

Yolanda was a lady of considerable elegance, and there she sat, immaculately dressed, with yesterday's newspaper on her lap. We were then each given a tray, one of those with a landscape painted on it, to put on top of our newspapers. Dinner consisted of roast lamb and vegetables and really was very good.

At one point while eating and half watching the

TV, a familiar sound and smell broke the tedium. One of the cats, Charlie I think they said his name was, had decided to use the half-full litter tray next to the couch, and sadly had more than a touch of diarrhoea. Yolanda gently put down her knife and fork and slowly closed her eyes. For her the dinner had pretty much ended. Phillip thought it was funny, but then Phillip thought many things were funny. I must admit, I had a bit of a chuckle, careful not to let Yolanda see me. It was more through disbelief than anything else. How could people live like this?

After this astonishing performance, Marlene said: "Tony, I wonder if you'd have a look at him? He's had that problem for some time now."

I swallowed my mouthful, and thought: "If you knew he had 'that problem', why didn't you put him outside during dinner?"

"Bring him into the hospital tomorrow," I suggested. "I'll be happy to have a look at him. I didn't bring anything with me."

Marlene then looked at Yolanda, who now had Charlie sitting right next to her on the couch.

"Aren't you hungry, dear?" she asked. "You've hardly touched your dinner. Don't you like it?"

"Oh no, it was delicious, really. It's just that I had a late lunch."

"Liar," I muttered under my breath.

Marlene was happy with that explanation. So too, apparently was Charlie, who was purring and licking the gravy from the edge of Yolanda's plate.

From time to time Charlie broke wind, which Phillip thought was pretty funny. Marlene seemed oblivious to the smell. Yolanda wasn't. She was sitting rigidly, the colour having disappeared from her cheeks.

The main course over, we had apple crumble and coffee.

After dinner I ventured into the somewhat rustic bathroom — situated appropriately, I thought, next to the kitchen — and had to persuade one cat off the toilet seat while two others watched me intently from their vantage point in the shower recess.

At around 8.30 I sensed Yolanda had had enough. I actually sensed she'd had enough around 4.30, so I politely thanked Marlene and Phillip for a wonderful evening, explaining that I wanted an early night as I had surgery the next morning.

As we left, and having trodden in something that didn't make it to the litter tray, Yolanda paused half way to the car and said quietly but firmly: "Don't you ever do that to me again. The next invitation by any of your clients and you're on your own."

It was the last of it she would ever mention. I felt I'd been let off lightly.

After six months the practices had become so busy that I'd been given an assistant, Toby, to help me handle the workload.

One of Toby's first patients was a dead budgie. At least, Toby knew it was dead — he hadn't realised that the bird's elderly owners thought it was merely lethargic.

When Toby said to them: "Take a seat. I'll take Bluey into the surgery for a moment and examine him," they had no idea he was going to do an autopsy. They thought he was going to work out some sort of treatment. So when he returned as chipper as can be with the results, they were stunned.

"What do you mean 'autopsy'?" the husband said.

"Surely you knew he was dead?" Toby asked, when he saw how catatonic the couple had become.

"No, we thought Bluey was still breathing."

"Not when I got him he wasn't." In this instance, Toby's bedside manner left a little to be desired.

The year Toby and I worked together was wonderful. I could extend the consulting hours at each place, as there was no need to be running frantically between them any more. We could also share the after-hours work, and so my social life and sleep patterns soon improved.

I wished we could have continued longer, but I started to notice worrying chinks in the management of the practices.

I couldn't convince Chris or Tim to buy various essential things, like extra cages or a second-hand X-ray machine for Pyrmont for the increasing workload. We were still transporting animals for X-rays, and the numbers of X-rays we were now taking made that ridiculous. And medical companies would no longer supply us unless the invoices were paid COD.

Apparently they hadn't been getting paid and huge debts had begun to mount. I couldn't understand how that could happen — we were so busy, I was sure our costs should have been covered. I had no idea where the money was going.

Whenever I approached Tim about it he would brush it aside with some glib bravado about how it wasn't a problem and that the various suppliers didn't know what they were talking about.

"That may be the case," I said. "But if none of them supply us, our standard of care is sure going to dip sharply."

Bank managers would also phone, but when I gave Tim those messages he would never return their calls either. So I found myself dealing with their grievances on a regular basis.

As much as I wanted to stay, I felt it was unwise to have my name associated with a history of bad debt.

I'd decided that it was as good a time as any to do what many twenty-five-year-old vet graduates do: head overseas and work in Britain for a while.

It's funny how, as we get older, our priorities change. And the awareness of these changes can be quite sudden and dramatic. Three years after leaving Tim and Chad's practice I woke up one morning in a youth hostel in Munich and thought to myself: "My God, you're nearly twenty-eight years old and you don't have anything. You don't have a car, you don't have a house, you don't have any money, and you don't have any plans." It was time to come home and set up a base.

It had probably been the best three years of my life — doing locums in England and Wales during the summer, skiing and living the high life in Aspen during the winter, and travelling around Europe in between — but, like all good things (as the cliché goes) it had to come to an end.

So, after a last tour through Europe, and that revelation in the Munich youth hostel, I headed home.

I was able to get a well-paid job fairly quickly in a Sydney practice, but after ten months I began to get itchy feet about having my own hospital.

Then out of the blue came a phone call.

"Hi, Tony. I heard you were back in town."

It was Tim Darkhome. I was intrigued as to why he'd be calling. I figured it wasn't just a belated welcome back into the country. He probably had some get-rich-quick scam he was going to offer me.

"Hi, Tim. What's up?"

"I was wondering if you'd like to work for me again — I'll give you ten per cent of the profits on top of your wage."

Judging by my last experience with Tim, I calculated ten per cent of nothing was always going to be nothing and so with a boldness that still amazes me I made a counter offer:

"No, Tim. Either sell me the whole thing, lock, stock and barrel, or forget it."

"All right. Let's have lunch and discuss the details."

It was that fast. Not a moment's hesitation or even some counter offer. He really must have needed money in a hurry. Obviously his business acumen hadn't improved much these past few years. I couldn't imagine how run-down the practices must have become. I found out his partnership with Chris had folded bitterly and Tim was left with the two practices that I used to manage. Chris had another two.

We met for lunch the following weekend and haggled over the price. As usual Tim ate and drank well. Then when the bill for lunch came he was again without his wallet. I paid. He said he'd pay me back. He never did. The more things change . . .

Not surprisingly, the deal fell through despite Tim's initial eagerness. While I was disappointed at first, in retrospect it was probably a godsend. Two practices, one in Glebe and one in Surry Hills, came up for same at around the same time, and I was able to buy them at a reasonable price. It was my chance to kick-start my career. I set about immediately refurbishing the hospitals and buying much-needed equipment.

Over the next few years I only heard rumours about what Tim was doing with his life. One was that he'd opened up another practice in the country, and it had folded. Another was that he'd become a horse consultant, and yet another that he was growing avocados and soy beans somewhere in the north of

Queensland. Apparently none of the ventures had done well.

Chris had apparently had to sell his two practices because he'd been deregistered by the Veterinary Surgeons Board for certain indiscretions. Subsequently he'd opened up a laundromat, which then burned down. After that, he drove a cab for a while, and later worked for an elevator company. What a sad fall from grace.

chapter 4

Cuddle Pie

I walked out into the waiting room and was talking to Martina as she typed information into the computer. As I bent forward to book in Mrs Johnson's Silkie Terrier for dental work, I heard ferocious growling. Turning my head slightly to the side, I saw a large German Shepherd baring his teeth and snarling at me menacingly.

"Who's that?" I whispered to Martina.

"That's Cuddle Pie Schneider," she said. "Cute, isn't he."

"His name's Cuddle Pie?"

"Yes, and he's next," Martina smirked.

I braced myself and picked up the relevant card.

"Go through to the surgery, Mr Schneider," I said to the stocky, blond Aryan who was struggling to hold back his "pet".

He held the lead tightly as Cuddle Pie tried to

launch himself at me as they walked past. Mr Schneider was laughing at this display of aggression. For some unknown reason there are people who think it's funny to have a dog that terrifies people.

Steeling myself, I walked into the consulting room. Staying close to the walls, I circled until I reached the other side of the examination table. Cuddle Pie's eyes followed me closely.

"So," I said, "what seems to be the problem?"

"It's his backside," Mr Schneider began to explain. "He's got these really deep, bleeding sores around his backside."

"Great," I thought despondently. "How the hell am I going to examine that?"

Keeping my distance I explained to Mr Schneider that German Shepherds can get a disease called anal furunculosis, which causes very deep and painful ulcerations around the rear end. These areas have to be curetted to get rid of all the infected tissue so healthy tissue can regrow.

"We're going to have to anaesthetise Cuddle Pie for this procedure," I said. "Has he eaten today?"

"Yes, about an hour before coming in."

"OK then, we'll have to do him tomorrow. Don't give him any breakfast and bring him back in the morning," I said, with some misgiving.

I gave Mr Schneider some sedatives for Cuddle Pie in the hope the dog would be a little settled when he next came in.

As Mr Schneider took Cuddle Pie out the front

door I turned to Martina and, with the dread of a man destined for the gallows, said: "He's coming in for surgery tomorrow."

Martina, ever the compassionate shoulder, said simply: "Well then, let the games begin."

She seemed to be looking forward to the clash. I couldn't understand how she could be so unworried. It wasn't as though she was going to be a passive spectator.

I didn't sleep well that night, anxious about my forthcoming Apocalypse.

The next morning came all too soon.

Cuddle Pie arrived and appeared fairly subdued. Martina took him by the lead and calmly led him into the kennel area. No sign of aggression, not the slightest hint of resistance. The sedatives had worked well. It was almost disappointing. What had I lost sleep for?

We tied him to a fitting on the wall, as we thought we might have difficulty getting him out of a cage, and I drew up a syringe with a sedative.

"OK, Martina," I said, "you hold the lead tight while I jab him."

She undid the lead and I proceeded to the non-biting end, and crouched to give the injection in the muscle of the back leg. The myth of Cuddle Pie's co-operation exploded violently. He turned and lunged at me in an instant, knocking me onto the seat of my pants. Martina managed to keep hold of his lead as I remained, stunned, on my rump.

"Christ!" I exclaimed, goggle-eyed. "What the hell was that?"

Cuddle Pie stood glaring at me, whereas Martina was laughing the laugh of one who had just survived death.

"Quick, isn't he?" she giggled nervously. And then, after a short pause: "What do we do now, Hercules?"

I got up, brushed myself off and, regaining my composure, considered the next option. "We go to Plan B."

"Really?" said Martina. "Was that just Plan A?"

I decided to ignore her cynicism. "Here's what we're going to have to do," I began, with a certain authority. This had now become personal. I didn't like to concede defeat in these situations and this beast was not going to get the better of me. "You grab him tightly and walk him slowly through the doorway. When he's half way through, I'll close the door so he can't move. Then I'll inject him. How does that sound?"

She looked at me disdainfully.

"Trust me on this one," I said. "Once I clamp the door shut, he won't be able to move."

Cuddle Pie obediently followed Martina through and I quickly closed the door. But the very second he felt trapped, his adrenaline made him invincible again. Martina held on determinedly, almost getting whiplash as Cuddle Pie exploded through the door. She wasn't about to let go of the lead, and once away from the doorway he settled again.

Martina's face was flushed and she was panting rapidly. "Plan C, doctor?"

It was obviously time to call in reinforcements. If my associate, Richard, had finished operating at the other hospital he could come over and give us a hand. I phoned him.

"We've got this dog over here that's a little bit stroppy."

Martina rolled her eyes. "And Hitler was a bit pushy," she mumbled.

Richard said he'd be over straight after lunch. He was never one to rush things, never one to be spurred into action unnecessarily. He arrived about forty-five minutes later, which gave us time to recharge our batteries.

"That's Cuddle Pie, Richard. We're onto Plan C," Martina explained.

"What happened to Plans A and B?"

"You don't want to know."

"I see," said Richard. "A bit anxious, is he?"

"Just a smidge," said Martina.

I was ready to resume the battle. "Here's what I reckon we ought to do," I said. "We'll put two leads around his neck and then, when I give the call, you two pull in different directions. That way he won't be able to turn and attack me when I hold his back leg and inject him from behind."

Plan C wasn't greeted with the overwhelming applause I thought it deserved. Richard and Martina just looked at each other sceptically. The failures of my previous efforts had left them less than optimistic.

We put the two leads on and, while Richard and Martina pulled tightly in opposite directions, I grabbed Cuddle Pie from behind. He was throwing his legs about frantically with me hanging on for dear life. By the time I managed to get the injection in I was on my back clinging to his leg. Triumphantly I looked up at the others and held up the empty syringe like a trophy.

Martina held up a clenched fist. "Yes!"

"Well done, Anthony," Richard said politely, in his usual subdued way.

Once Cuddle Pie was heavily sedated we were able to fully anaesthetise him and curette the area.

The trouble with anal furunculosis was that it could recur, and I had warned Mr Schneider of this prior to surgery.

Later that day he came to pick up Cuddle Pie. "How was he, doctor?"

"No trouble," I said matter-of-factly, to complete my victory. I wasn't going to give him the satisfaction. "Everything went well. We will, however, have to see Cuddle Pie for a check-up."

Martina looked at me, completely mystified, and mouthed the words: "Are you kidding?"

Cuddle Pie came back for a check-up two weeks later. His lesions healed fairly well over time, although they never entirely disappeared. His temperament, however, never improved. He bit through the finger of a relieving vet who foolishly had said she could handle him, despite having been warned to be careful. She went home with her hand in bandages.

Eventually we had to refer Cuddle Pie to the Sydney University Veterinary Hospital as his problem had recurred. There the staff had to perform a radical surgery to try and permanently alleviate the condition. They phoned me after seeing Cuddle Pie and told me that, because he was dangerous, they had suggested euthanasia. After that we never saw Cuddle Pie again, although we know Mr Schneider refused their offer.

chapter 5

The trouble with Harvey

I first met Harvey Gresham on a dismally cold July afternoon.

"Hello, that the vet? Miss Gresham here." It was a powerful voice that bellowed into the phone. "My Harvey's not lookin' too well. Sneezing and coughing, the whole bit. I was wondering if you could pop by and have a look at him. It's a bit chilly to get him down to you today."

Being such a bitterly cold day we weren't too busy and so it was no problem to fit in a home visit.

"That'll be no problem," I replied. "How's 2.30 this afternoon suit you?"

"Wonderful!" she roared. "I'll see you then."

Miss Gladys Gresham almost never spoke softly. At first I thought she must have had a hearing problem. But she turned out to be one of those people who just have the volume switch turned up higher than the rest of us. Usually those sort of people really aggravate me. I regard it as arrogance that they think everyone within earshot is interested in what they have to say. But Miss Gresham was different. She was certainly raucous, definitely rough around the edges, but one would be lucky to find a more genuine and loving person. In her it wasn't abrasive.

She was a large woman, in her late thirties or early forties, I suppose. Her hair was short and dyed jet black with a fringe about one inch from the eyebrows. This accentuated the roundness of her face and the redness of her generous cheeks.

I arrived at her flat, one of three on the ground floor of a fairly unimaginative red brick building only about five minutes from the hospital. It was a three-storey government block whose landscaping consisted only of mowed lawn surrounds. No flowers or shrubs anywhere.

Miss Gresham answered the door. "Good to see you. Come in. Come in. The patient's over there."

On this day she wore a yellow T-shirt with a picture of a flexed biceps on the back, baggy red trousers and a pair of blue thongs. Quite a fashion statement. She was like that. Dressed for comfort.

The flat itself was very small. A green Laminex table occupied the centre of the lounge-cum-dining room. A two-seater sofa sat under a window shaded by Venetian blinds, with two single chairs on the other side of the room. A tiny kitchen joined the lounge room. Once a stove, fridge and sink had been somehow squeezed in there seemed little room for anything else. I wondered how Miss Gresham managed to move around in it.

And amid all these fairly basic suburban furnishings were the wall decorations. There was one standard landscape but the predominant artworks, if that's what you could call them, were photographs of young men in varying stages of undress. Not full frontals, more the type of thing one would see in body building magazines: massive sweaty backs and pectorals, and the odd flexed buttock. Who would have thought? This chunky, unremarkable woman had a fetish. People are sometimes hard to pick. The exterior is obviously not always a reflection of what's going on inside. It was difficult to conceal a smile as I looked around.

I dragged my attention from the decor.

"Let's have a look at Harvey, then," I said, redirecting my focus.

He was sitting on the sofa under the window. He was an enormous Siamese male. Not so much obese, although he was carrying some excess baggage, he was just a huge cat. He sat in a pool of sunlight that entered through the window in the afternoon. Cats are all born with a sunlight magnet. They have to seek it out and luxuriously bask in it or they perish. His eyes hovered in that limbo area between being asleep and awake. He didn't seem in the least perturbed by my presence. But that, I was to learn, was Harvey. Nothing bothered him. He was the definition of laid back.

"Big isn't he?" I said, stating the obvious. Miss Gresham must have been sick of people making that gem of a perception. "How old is he?"

"He's about twelve years old now, I think. Been a great mate over the years. He really hasn't eaten much the last few days."

I examined Harvey, who was totally unconcerned by my prodding and probing. Even the thermometer was accepted without objection. He was running a fever and was very snuffly. His eyes were weeping and he would have frequent sneezing attacks. Poor old Harvey had the 'flu.

I gave him an injection to bring down his fever and an antibiotic. Miss Gresham was to continue antibiotics for the next five days.

"If he's not showing any improvement in the next couple of days, let me know," I instructed as I left.

With that she saw me out with a powerful whack on the back. If I'd had a mouthguard I would have spat it out.

"You do worry about the little buggers don't you?" she bellowed.

Two days later she phoned to tell me Harvey was feeling a whole lot better.

"Just thought you'd like to know. You did a great job on him."

The last bit made me feel like a carpenter, but it is always gratifying when people let you know if treatments have been successful. They certainly let you know if they haven't.

It had been quite some time before I heard from Miss Gresham again. It was a sunny summer's day and so she was able to bring Harvey to the hospital. They arrived during the morning consultation period. Harvey was in his blue plastic basket, which he almost completely filled. It was strapped to her shopping trolley and, as always, his demeanour was calm. Harvey travelled well.

"Come in, Miss Gresham," I motioned. "What's up with Harvey?"

"He's drinking an awful lot of water, Mr Sheldon, an awful lot," she said, with what I perceived as more than a little concern. But then to minimise the appearance of her anxiety she continued with her usual chuckle, "Just water though, not like me."

"Has his appetite been OK?" I asked.

"Can't fill him up. He's always hungry. I know he's big but honestly, he's never been a real big eater, even a bit fussy at times. Now he'll eat just about anything, even vegetables. He'd never touch them before. I left a huge piece of rump out on the kitchen sink the other day and he ate the whole damn thing. He's driving me crazy."

I wasn't happy with the sound of all that and asked if I could keep Harvey for the day to run some tests.

She patted Harvey and explained the situation to him. "Now listen, mate, you have to stay here for the day with Mr Sheldon so he can make you better. I'll come back for you this evening."

I took some blood and the results confirmed my concern that Harvey had become diabetic. It was much rarer in cats than dogs and harder to stabilise as they couldn't always be relied upon to eat at the right time. It meant that Harvey would have to be given insulin injections twice daily and I wasn't sure how Miss Gresham would accept that. Because she seemed to be a "call a spade a spade" type of person I felt her attitude would be: he's had a bloody good life up till now, and he's not young, so it might be best to declare his innings and put him to sleep.

Most people opted for that choice. Keeping a stabilised diabetic animal can be a chore at the best of times.

"Miss Gresham, won't you come in. I'd like to have a chat to you about Harvey. Have a seat."

"Sounds a bit ominous," she said, pulling up a chair and putting Harvey on her lap. "What's the verdict, doc?"

"Well, Harvey has diabetes."

"You mean like in people?" She laughed, albeit a little nervously. Then she grabbed Harvey's head in her hands and looked straight at him. "You silly old bugger."

I explained to her there were only two choices. She could either decide to let us stabilise him in hospital and then continue to give him insulin at home. Or, if not, then it would be better to have him put down.

"I don't know," she mumbled, continually stroking Harvey's back. "I just don't know. He is old. What do you reckon?"

I suggested he was very fit for his age, but that it was a commitment that couldn't be taken lightly. If the procedures weren't adhered to strictly and consistently it could lead to unnecessary suffering for Harvey. I recommended she go home and have a hard think about it.

"No," she answered quickly, the bravado returning to her voice. "He's my little mate, and so you gotta give him a chance don't you?" Then she looked at Harvey. "You silly old flip. That was a stupid thing to go and get now, wasn't it?"

Harvey spent the next five days in hospital having his insulin dosage stabilised. On his discharge we had to instruct Miss Gresham how to give injections. Initially, as with most people, she was apprehensive with a hypodermic syringe in her hand. She shook as she tried to give Harvey an injection. But he was so patient. She tried a few times before she got it right, but insulin needles being so fine he seemed almost totally oblivious to them. Pretty soon she had it down pat. I felt Harvey was lucky to have her and would probably do well.

"We're going to do just fine, Mr Sheldon," she laughed as she wheeled him out.

For the first few months Harvey would come in for regular blood sugar tests to monitor the success of his treatment at home. They were always pretty normal and he looked a picture of health. Harvey and I got to know each other quite well over the years. We became pretty close. He always seemed pleased to see me even though I'm sure taking a blood sample wasn't pleasant. Of course you wouldn't know with Harvey. He purred through the whole thing anyway. And when it was over he'd stick out his chin to be patted underneath it. That, I was told, was his favourite thing. And if you did that while he lay in his patch of sunlight he was transported to another even higher plane of pleasure.

"He doesn't mind his injections at all. Must know he's going to get something to eat a bit later." Miss Gresham was her usual ebullient self. "We're a great little team, aren't we, Harve?"

Because the two of them were doing so well I decided to make the blood tests less frequent. We agreed on every three months.

I don't know what transpired over the next several months, but somewhere along the way Miss Gresham found God. She came in with Harvey for his next test and as usual the results were perfect. Then she told me how she had gone to the Town Hall with a friend who'd asked her to listen to "some preacher bloke" give a sermon. She wasn't much into that sort of thing, she said. Thought it was all a bit of hocus-pocus and only went along to keep her friend company. And then, apparently at this sermon, a miracle had occurred. Her back trouble had somehow been cured. And so she had become a born-again

Christian. Miss Gresham didn't seem the type taken by miracles and religious rhetoric. But the best was yet to come. She went on to describe a religious experience she'd had with Harvey one evening.

"You know, Mr Sheldon, I was watching this preacher fella on the television, you know, the one who cured my back at the Town Hall. He was giving another sermon and I held Harvey's paws up to the screen and he was cured too. It was another bloody miracle."

I tried to picture the scene. It was too bizarre. This amazing, religious happening with quivering cat's paws, television sets, impassioned evangelists, and all presided over by a huge picture of some bodybuilder's sweaty rear end. But Harvey was cool. He would have been in anything without complaint.

"What do you mean cured? You're still giving him the insulin aren't you?" I asked, beginning to feel uncomfortable about this holy revelation.

"Oh yeah, he still gets that." Then after a short pause she asked: "I wonder if you'd write an article for our Christian magazine about Harvey's miracle cure?"

I thought I was a pretty good judge of people but this sudden devoutness certainly came out of nowhere. From walls full of sweaty nude men to pious Christianity was a quantum leap. And I wondered what constituted a cure in her mind if she was still giving him the insulin anyway.

I said I couldn't honestly write that article unless Harvey was able to survive without his insulin and I wasn't willing to test that. Miss Gresham, with all her new-found faith was, thankfully, unwilling to risk it either, but steadfastly maintained her belief that he was cured.

I'd learnt over the years not to debate clients' personal religious beliefs even if their connection with logic was breathtakingly thin. What was important here was that Harvey's health wasn't being compromised.

Miss Gresham, holding both my hands in hers, looking into my eyes and smiling the way only evangelical people can, told me she understood. That was good because I didn't.

Thankfully she maintained her visits fairly regularly and kept up the insulin. Harvey had by now been a successful diabetic for about three years. His last check-up had been about five months ago but now, on this visit, I was surprised. He'd lost so much weight. He didn't look like the Harvey I knew. I could feel his ribs, and his face, once round and handsome, was now thinner and more angular. He still put his chin out to be scratched.

"He still gets his insulin regularly, Mr Sheldon, but he's getting so damn thin. And he's drinking an awful lot of water again, just like before."

We tested his blood sugar again and it was normal. Unfortunately, at fifteen, age had finally caught up with Harvey Gresham. Further testing diagnosed him as being in severe kidney failure. His blood sugar levels were irreversibly and unsustainably high.

"I think this might be the end of the road for him," I confided grimly. "His kidneys are gone. We could put him on a drip for a couple of days and he'd be great for a short time but then he'd quickly deteriorate again."

I believe she had already realised Harvey's fate when she brought him in. I only confirmed it.

"That's it then, isn't it?" she said sadly.

"I'm afraid it is."

"Then it's best we let him go, Mr Sheldon. I don't want to put him through any more. He looks so unhappy."

I asked her, as I ask all people in this situation, if they'd like to be with their pet while he was being put to sleep.

"Oh no, I couldn't watch that. I'll just say my goodbyes now."

And with a quiet dignity that somehow didn't surprise me despite the gruff exterior, Miss Gresham held Harvey in her arms and, with tears running down her face, patted him for the last time. "See you, mate. We'll get together again some day."

She left the surgery with the empty cat basket on her trolley and we sent the little trouper on his way. It was one of the hardest things I've ever had to do.

We never saw or heard from Miss Gresham again.

chapter 6

The pyramid

Mark Bentley rushed into the hospital in a panic, carrying his Kelpie in his arms. "My dog's just been hit by a car!"

"Go straight through," Eliza directed. Everyone in the waiting room also motioned him to go ahead.

Mr Bentley came into the consulting room, sweating profusely, his face white with shock, his eyes wide with disbelief. He was probably in his mid twenties, and wore one of those open-necked painted-looking shirts, faded torn jeans and bare feet. He had an earring on his left ear and one of those peace signs that look like a Mercedes-Benz-emblem-gone-wrong around his neck. And, despite the fact he looked like he didn't have a brass razoo, he carried a mobile phone in his back pocket.

"Put him on the table gently," I instructed. "Now let's see what sort of damage we've done."

"I should have had him on a lead. I should have had him on a lead."

He was right of course, but this was hardly the time for a lecture.

"Do you think he'll be all right, doctor?"

"I don't know just yet," I answered. "It's much too early to tell."

It was a common question most people asked immediately following a car accident, and one that, in severe trauma cases like this one, I had difficulty answering. I didn't like the fact that there was no feeling in any of the Kelpie's legs and that he could only move his head and nothing else. I pinched his toes and got no response. Clamped artery forceps to the tip of his tail. Nothing. It didn't look good. There was a chance it could have been just spinal shock and he'd be OK in the morning, but I doubted it.

"We're going to have to X-ray him. I think he may have broken his neck." There is no easy way of saying something like that.

"Oh sh——!" Mr Bentley responded eloquently. "Jesus!" He stroked his dog while intermittently grumbling various profanities of dismay and self-blame. "God! I'm sorry, Kelly. It's all my fault."

Mr Bentley looked up towards me, child-like. "What if it is broken? Can it be fixed?"

"That depends," I said. "If the spinal cord is in one piece then it could just be severe bruising and we may have a chance, but if it is cut in two then there's nothing we can do."

"Jesus!"

"Pop back in this evening and we'll talk about the results of his X-rays. There's nothing else you can do now."

Mr Bentley left the hospital dejected. I wished I could have given a more optimistic outlook but realistically Kelly's condition looked awful. People in the waiting room, sensing his grief, tried to bolster his spirits with "Don't worry, he'll be OK," and "They're very good here, he's in good hands."

As I continued to examine Kelly on the table, Eliza walked in. "How bad is he?"

"I don't think he's got a hope in hell," I said honestly.

The X-rays confirmed the worst. The spinal cord was broken in half and displaced. I wasn't looking forward to telling Mr Bentley. I was sure his grieving was going to be loud. But sometimes people react very differently to how you would have expected. Mr Bentley was about to surprise me.

When he came back that evening, still looking totally miserable, he sat in the waiting room, head bowed, just staring at the floor.

"Come in, Mr Bentley," I said. "I'd like to show you Kelly's X-rays."

"It's bad news, isn't it?" he said, his hands in his pockets, his gaze unfocused but directed towards the X-rays.

"I'm afraid it is." I pointed out the damaged area on the radiograph. "Sadly, there's nothing we can do for him. As you can see, his spinal cord is cut completely in half."

I don't think Mr Bentley saw anything.

The events that were about to ensue were as strange, and in retrospect as tragic, as any I would ever see in my veterinary career.

There was a period of silence as he stared blankly ahead.

"Can he travel by car?" Mr Bentley asked, still staring.

"Can he what?" Perhaps I'd heard incorrectly.

"Can I take him in the car?" he repeated. "Out to the country?"

So startling was the question, I felt like saying: "Yes, like a surfboard, on roof racks, as long as you don't pull the ockie straps too tight." But I sensed Mr Bentley may have been serious — and this was certainly no time to be flippant — so I asked what I felt under the circumstances was a fairly reasonable question: "Why?"

His answer reaffirmed my belief that, no matter what you may have seen or heard before, you can still be totally astonished.

"I'd like to take Kelly out to the country and build a Perspex pyramid and put him under it," he explained with some new-found optimism.

I suppose I should have suspected something, with that peace-and-love thing around his neck. I again ventured forth with what I thought was another reasonable question: "Why?"

"Well," he went on, "I want to put a whole lot of crystals around the pyramid and that will draw negative ions into it and into Kelly, and that might help him recover."

Sound medical logic, I thought.

"But two parts of his spinal cord are nowhere near each other. That's a fair sort of structural deficit for negative ions to works on," I suggested.

I wasn't against all forms of alternative medicine; many have their place. But all things considered, I felt that the efficacy of negative ions in this case was going to be somewhat marginal.

"Negative ions can do incredible things," he confidently asserted, the colour returning to his cheeks.

But I knew what I knew, and Mr Bentley was heading for a fall. Desperation can make fools of us all.

"I'm sure they can, but I'd like you to take some of these pain killers with you in case your therapy doesn't work and Kelly becomes uncomfortable. And if it all gets too much for him you must bring him back so we can end any further suffering."

To this day I wish I'd forbidden Mr Bentley from pursuing this crazy venture, but I was young and inexperienced and didn't have the confidence to veto it. Today it would be so much easier. I would just say: "Don't be so ridiculous. You can't fix a broken neck with a pyramid!" And that would have been the end of it, right there.

So Mr Bentley gently carried Kelly out to his Mini-Moke for their journey of faith.

A little curious as to why they were leaving the hospital together, Eliza asked: "Where's he going?"

"He's going out to the country to put his dog under a pyramid. Then he's going to throw crystals all around it. That way all the negative ions can fix Kelly's neck."

"Really?" Eliza replied, closing her eyes in disgust. "That ought to work."

Two days later the phone call came. "I don't think this is working, doctor." Mr Bentley's voice was soft and trembling. He was calling on his mobile phone, out by his tribute to Egypt.

"Kelly's not moving at all?" I asked, knowing full well the answer.

"No, he hasn't responded," came the dejected reply.

"Well, you gave it your best shot. Don't be too hard on yourself."

"Maybe the injury was too great, and I don't think the crystals I bought were all that good either."

"Yes, I've heard some are better than others."

It was time to end this foolishness, however well intentioned it may have been.

"Well then, bring Kelly back. No point in dragging it out any further. I think it's time to put an end to his suffering."

Having his almost inaudible approval, I hung up the phone.

"Eliza," I called out. "That was Mr Bentley. The pyramid didn't work."

"Is that right? How come?"

"Faulty crystals."

Mr Bentley came in that evening, understandably shattered and probably a little embarrassed.

"Do you think I did the wrong thing?"

"You did what you thought was right."

He stayed with Kelly while we put him to sleep and then took him back out to the country, this time to rest more peacefully.

chapter 7

Skin deep

Mr and Mrs Stanton had two Staffordshire Bull Terriers, Theo and Tanya. Theo was aggressive. He bit everyone. He bit their children, he bit the gardener, and he bit the builder when he tried to climb down from his ladder. We'd tried everything to reduce his aggression. We desexed him and that didn't work. We tried hormonal therapy and that didn't work. We tried instilling discipline — his rebelling against that almost made it worse. Finally the Stanton family, reluctantly, but with my full support, agreed enough was enough. Someone was going to get seriously hurt, and so we sent Theo on his final journey.

That left Tanya, lovable, scatty Tanya. She wasn't the smartest dog in the world. She had an attention span of about two and a half seconds, and the concentration of an amoeba. But Tanya had love and affection to burn. She loved the kids, loved the gardener, and the builder spent much less time stranded up his ladder.

One evening Mrs Stanton brought Tanya to the hospital with a large cut on her forehead. It was a gaping wound some five centimetres long and two centimetres wide, leaving a constant stream of blood running down the middle of her nose.

Tanya, of course, was totally unmoved.

"I don't know how she did it," Mrs Stanton said. "Doesn't she look dreadful?"

I somehow got the feeling that aesthetics were largely at issue here.

Mrs Stanton was a young mother of four children. Her husband was a businessman on the board of some big corporation. They lived in one of the more affluent suburbs of Sydney and wanted only the best for their pets. They were the type of client every vet loves — caring people with the means to pursue any diagnostic or surgical procedure necessary. It's rewarding to be able to follow a case through fully and so reduce the level of guesswork. Unfortunately, many people are unable to afford that luxury.

I examined the wound closely.

"I think it looks worse than it is," I said. "It's only skin deep. We should be able to get the edges together fairly well."

"Can you do it so there isn't a scar?"

My hunch about the aesthetics priority was right.

"Well, it can be done almost invisibly," I explained.

"We use very fine dissolvable sutures under the skin and very close to the wound edges. That brings those edges so close together that there is no need for external skin sutures and so scarring is minimised. However, it's vital to keep the wound dry, or those dissolving stitches will expand, loosen and the wound will reopen."

"Oh yes, let's do it that way," Mrs Stanton said, with a little too much gusto.

Suddenly I had a bad feeling about this. It worries me when such decisions are made without a second's hesitation. Risks always warrant at least a moment's thought, but here they were given none. It made me think that perhaps everything I'd said hadn't really sunk in. It seemed that the instant I'd said "no skin sutures" and "minimal scarring", any other consideration ended. Mrs Stanton's primary concern was that Tanya would remain aesthetically unflawed.

Having agreed to the "scar-free" option, Mrs Stanton brought Tanya into the hospital for surgery.

Once the dog was anaesthetised I carefully brought the skin edges together from underneath and finished what I considered a good job. You could hardly see where the wound had been.

Mrs Stanton returned that evening to pick up Tanya and was well pleased with the result.

"Gee, it looks terrific. You should have been a plastic surgeon," Mrs Stanton said, perhaps with some knowledge on the subject. "Tanya, aren't you still just the prettiest girl."

This preoccupation with glamour was a little unnerving. I had to interrupt the rapture between these two ladies to re-emphasise the critical point.

"Remember now, don't get her forehead wet. It's really important. I can't stress that too strongly."

"I won't, I won't," Mrs Stanton said, almost as a reflex, while hugging and kissing Tanya, who was jumping all over her with the joy of a long-lost relative. Mrs Stanton's reassurance was less than convincing.

"You really can't see anything," she repeated with amazement.

They left the surgery together, with Tanya continually jumping up at her beaming mother. Somehow I sensed that this episode wasn't over.

Three days later I had the 'flu. I'd worked all day with it and that night had put myself to bed with a fever and what I felt was an acceptable dose of self pity. It wasn't my turn to be on call and so I felt justifiably confident that after an uninterrupted night's sleep I would have a healthy return to work the next morning.

My father and brother, Mark, came over to see how I was doing, and brought with them some chicken soup from Mum. Do I believe that old Yiddish panacea really works? I know it doesn't hurt.

Mark strolled into my bedroom with his standard greeting for pretty much any occasion: "G'day, how's it going?" Even when I awoke in intensive care following surgery to correct a skull fracture which had led to meningitis, Mark was there with: "G'day, how's it going?" Consistency is a valuable asset in a family.

Dad came in with his standard greeting: "Hi, Shtern. What's up?" (Shtern being short for Shternen, his nickname for me, the origins of which I have no idea.) From broken limbs to broken romances, when I came to Dad for advice or needed pepping up, it was always: "Hi, Shtern. What's up?"

Mum's cooking was also dependable. At any time you could drop by and there'd be a feast in minutes. Not just a Vegemite sandwich but a banquet. And her reasons were always the same: "You know I love to cook" and "There's always so much food in the house, I hate to throw it out" (as if she would) and my favourite, "It's just something I put together with leftovers."

So here I was, sick and wallowing in congested misery, when in walks "G'day, how's it going?" and "Hi Shtern. What's up?" and the greatest chicken soup ever made. Consistency comforted me like a cocoon. A good night's sleep and I'd be better by morning for sure.

As welcome as it was, their stay was thankfully brief. Clogged up and feverish, I finally nodded off.

Then the damn phone rang. It jolted me upright like an electric cattle prod. I looked at the clock. It was 11.30. Who could possibly be ringing now? I decided to let it keep ringing until the caller got sick of it, and then I could go back to sleep. But it just kept ringing, a dozen or more times. Who could be that persistent?

Finally, having lost the war of attrition, I climbed

out of bed and walked dizzily to the telephone.

"Hello?" I mumbled, overly accentuating my congestion. Whoever it was should be in no doubt they had woken a very unwell young man.

"Hello, it's Mrs Stanton here. I'm so glad you're home."

Where else would I be near midnight on a Tuesday night?

"Tanya's been running through the sprinkler. Her head's soaking wet and the stitches have pulled apart. The wound is wide open again."

Why didn't that surprise me?

"Did you ring the hospital and get the after-hours emergency number?" I asked. I then coughed excessively, and sniffed a few times for good measure. But this elaborate 'flu performance was having no effect.

"Yes, but they wouldn't give me your number, so I looked it up in the phone book."

I thought I'd been pretty convincing with my near-death act, but she was either totally unaware or unconcerned that I was sick.

I decided to be blunt. "I'm actually in bed with a really bad 'flu."

"Well, what am I supposed to do?"

Bingo! Jackpot! Three lemons! I took a deep breath and clenched my jaw. "Would you like me to have a look at Tanya now?" I knew that was a stupid question.

"Oh, yes! Would you?"

"OK, I'll meet you at the hospital in about fifteen minutes." Then, for an added theatrical touch: "Do you mind if I stay in my pyjamas? I really don't feel like changing."

"Of course not."

I didn't think she'd mind. Mrs Stanton was generous to a fault.

So I left home in striped flannelette pyjamas, dressing gown, ug boots and headache. I arrived at the hospital suitably snotty.

Tanya's head had opened up nicely. It wasn't bleeding but you could see frayed, wet suture ends hanging over the edges.

"Can I leave her with you? She looks terrible again doesn't she?"

I was in no mood now to debate the cosmetic angle. "This time, Mrs Stanton, I'm going to have to put proper skin sutures in," I said firmly. "Tanya's obviously not sensible enough to stay out of the water, is she?"

"No, she's not." Mrs Stanton seemed totally unfazed by the fact that I looked straight at her when I'd spoken of Tanya's lack of sense.

Left alone with Tanya, who I really was very fond of, I trudged into the operating theatre, hitched up my pyjama pants, tightened the dressing-gown cord and organised my instruments for surgery, all the time thinking how nice it would be to still be in bed.

I donned a surgical gown and began to restitch the wound. My nose was dripping continually. I thought of wearing a surgical mask, but the thought of sneezing into one of those put me off the idea. I used my sleeve.

I waited at the hospital until Tanya had woken sufficiently for it to be safe for me to go. I then drove home and lapsed into a three-hour coma before the alarm went off.

I arrived at the hospital next morning looking like death. I should have brushed my hair.

"Boy, you must have had a good night," Martina said with a sly leer.

I will never understand why, when you look like a half-drowned sewer rat in the morning, everyone thinks you must have had a great night.

"By the way, there's a lady in the waiting room with a cake for you," Martina added, winking suggestively.

I ignored her. I wasn't in the mood.

I walked into the waiting room and there was Mrs Stanton. "I'm so sorry about getting you out of bed last night. I was just so very worried about Tanya."

She gave me the cake — a huge Black Forest cake, which in my state of semi-conscious queasiness was the last thing I felt like eating. For the first time in this whole incident, she was looking a little embarrassed. "I really am sorry."

As usual, I weakened. "That's OK," I said with a snuffle and a smile. "I'll just leave my phone off the hook tonight."

I have since had a silent number installed.

chapter 8

Bedside manner

I walked up the steep, narrow, dingy stairs that led to Gwen Smith's inner-city apartment. They smelt damp and mouldy, like a wet towel that had been left in the boot of your car too long. Gwen's was the only flat on the second floor of a little, run-down two-storey building, made even more glum by the flaking paint of the dark green exterior. It hadn't been an easy place to find. Situated toward the end of a narrow dead-end street, it was almost completely engulfed by surrounding high-rise industrial complexes. Very little light got through those factories to street level, and even now at two in the afternoon it was dim and bleak. This was mugging territory.

I was half way up the stairs leading to her front door when I heard the door of the ground-floor unit open with an eerie creak. I looked around. Standing in the doorway, staring at me, was a fat sweaty man in a dirty white singlet, blue shorts and thongs. The shorts were far too tight and riding up the insides of his thighs. He had oily, short black semi-balding hair and a monstrous double chin that hadn't seen a razor for days. The hallway lamp above his door highlighted the droplets of sweat on his head, neck and hairy shoulders. He just stood there, chewing on his Chiko roll, only stopping to periodically snort nasally and swallow.

It seemed like the Missing Link and I had been staring at each other for ages, suspended in time, although I'm sure it was probably only a few seconds. I was somehow mesmerised by his revoltingness. After thousands of years of evolution and huge advances in medical research, this was the legacy of Darwin's "survival of the fittest"? I consoled myself with the thought that he must have been the result of some horrendous genetic mutation that had somehow escaped the culling effects of "natural selection".

Finally dragging my attention from him I turned back up the stairs and continued the trek to Gwen's front door, a door cluttered with miscellaneous cat trinkets — ceramic cats, cat postcards and furry little cats randomly stuck all over it.

I knocked — using the cat-shaped door knocker — and soon she opened.

"Hi, love." She was smoking what I was soon to recognise as the almost everpresent cigarette. "Come in."

Gwen was probably in her late forties. She had

that world-weary look of having seen and done it all. Her eyes lacked sparkle, her skin was dull, and her breathing was somewhat laboured by all her years on the weed. But beneath this seemingly emotionless exterior lay an obvious love for her pets. Perhaps they'd given her less pain than the people who had passed fleetingly in and out of her life.

Only one step in and my eyes started to water uncontrollably from all the smoke. The whole interior was shrouded in a surreal haze. It was such a tiny apartment, a bedsitter really, and the ventilation was poor. The smoke was thicker than the worst pub I'd ever been in.

The kitchen was minuscule, hardly big enough to turn around in, and completely cluttered with dishes, a million other kitchen utensils, both washed and unwashed, and half-filled bowls of cat food.

The only other room was the all-in-one bedroom, dining room and television room. It was just as cluttered as the kitchen, with pillows, numerous full ashtrays, a couple of chairs and various articles of clothing spread randomly throughout the place. I never saw a bathroom in all the time I visited there, but I'm sure there must have been one hidden somewhere.

Apart from the stifling cigarette smog, the most overwhelming characteristic was the accumulation of hundreds of different cat ornaments. There were cat things everywhere, from fridge magnets to coasters, to paintings, posters, ceramics, stuffed toys and calendars. You couldn't look anywhere without being bombarded by images of cats.

Gwen had only three cats of her own and a fourteen-year-old Fox Terrier called Spot, so named because, unsurprisingly, of a spot over his right eye. They all lived snugly together, and despite the apparent anarchy of their home, it never smelt, at least not of animal excreta. Gwen was obviously careful to keep litter trays clean and give old Spot regular walks. Either that or the smoke just overwhelmed all the other smells.

On this particular visit, my first, I was to look at Smudge, her black male tomcat. He was troubled by a skin condition.

"Where would you like me to look at him?" I asked. There didn't seem enough room anywhere for a decent examination.

"On the edge of the bed should be fine," Gwen said.

So we both sat on the edge of the bed as I looked over old Smudge's scabby coat while she held him. As I parted his fur to see the type and extent of the lesions, I felt something pushing up against my backside. I turned around. There was a man in the bed!

"Did you know there was a man in your bed?" I asked Gwen.

"Yeah, that's Ken. He does shiftwork."

Well, I thought he was shifting a bit too close to me. I don't know how I missed noticing him or even sitting on him, but the bed was awash with clothing and pillows which were almost completely covering him. And he had been pushed up against the wall initially.

I now moved a little closer to the edge of the bed and continued my work with Smudge. Concentrating on the job at hand and trying to act like nothing here was unusual was difficult — Ken had now started to snore, with the odd guttural splutter thrown in for good measure. Gwen meanwhile had lit up another cigarette and was puffing frantically in my face. I was fighting both a desperate urge to cough and a feeling I was about to be sick. I somehow managed to resist both and get on with the examination.

Smudge had an allergic skin problem, caused primarily by fleas of which he had more than his fair share. There were fleas running all over him, masses of flea dirt all through his coat. I treated him for his irritation and suggested a regime which would control the fleas on all her pets as well as in their environment. They were all badly afflicted.

"Could you also have a look at Spot while you're here?" Gwen asked. "He seems to be having trouble chewing. He's hungry enough but keeps dropping the food out of his mouth like it hurts or something."

"Sure, pop him up. It sounds like it might be his teeth."

She lifted the little fellow up off the floor and put him on my lap. He seemed friendly enough, wagging his tail, and allowing me to pat him.

"OK, Spot. Let's have a look at that mouth of yours."

Then as I went to open it, quick as a flash, he savaged me. Tore into my hand like a frenzied maniac. Startled, I pulled my hand away quickly and accidentally smacked the sleeping Ken in the face. He opened his eyes in shock although I'm not sure he actually woke up, because he just as quickly rolled over and went back to sleep.

"He hates anyone looking at his mouth," Gwen informed me, five seconds too late.

I looked at my trembling hand. He'd drawn blood. It smelt like a sewer. I could only imagine what his teeth must be like.

"I'll have to take him with me to the hospital and clean those teeth under general anaesthetic," I explained. "I'll bring him back tomorrow."

"OK, love," she replied with her adenoidal twang.

I slowly and carefully got up from the bed with a once again calm Spot in hand, and being mindful not to wake Ken. It was a ridiculous precaution considering my not insignificant backhander had only momentarily startled him. That shiftwork must really knock you around.

Back at the hospital we anaesthetised Spot to get a better look at those teeth. Because of his age we had to be careful with the anaesthetic, and thankfully he got through it without too many problems. His teeth were putrid. They'd obviously had little attention at any time during his life. I cleaned and polished those that were salvageable and extracted the rest, which came to about eight. He slept off the anaesthetic at the hospital and I drove him home the next day.

As I walked into Gwen's building Neanderthal Man on the ground floor again opened his door and stared. He had on the same singlet, now with a few new tomato sauce stains down the front, the same neatly fitting shorts, and probably the same sweat. Only this time he was eating a meat pie and had a cigarette hanging off his bottom lip. I didn't want to imagine how he managed to combine the two. The man was fermenting.

I couldn't understand what he saw in me that was so fascinating. He obviously had a great deal of time on his hands and very little constructive activity with which to fill it.

I felt like asking him, "What is the attraction? What's so fascinating?" But I thought the better of it and silently continued past him, up the dark stairs.

"Hi, love," Gwen greeted me as she opened her door. "How is he?"

Her adenoids hadn't improved. Nor had the smog level. My eyes immediately began watering.

"He's fine, but I had to take a fair few teeth out because they were really bad. Try and get him to chew on some raw bones to help maintain those that he has left."

Across the room Ken was asleep again. I couldn't actually see him except for a bit of hair poking out the top of the blankets. But I could hear the snoring.

Gwen sat on the edge of the bed and cuddled Spot. I pulled up a sort of beanbag next to the bed.

"His mouth doesn't smell nearly so bad," Gwen said, as she held him up in front of her face.

Despite her monotone voice and somewhat hard exterior she really did love her animals, almost to the point of obsession. I knew that whatever instructions were given she would do her very best to carry them out to the letter.

I got up to leave but I couldn't contain my curiosity. "Who's the guy in the unit downstairs?"

"That's the landlord," Gwen answered. "He's a real pig!"

Literally or figuratively, I wondered.

"He always has to know who's coming and going," she went on enthusiastically. "A real busybody he is. I never tell him though. It's none of his business. I don't think he likes me having these animals here but he's a bigger bloody animal than any of the ones I've got."

"He does seem a bit unsightly, doesn't he?"

"Unsightly? He's a filthy swine. I don't think he's ever had a wash. Wouldn't know what a shower and a cake of soap looked like. And my God he stinks. You must have smelt him when you came in."

"It did seem a little stuffy I suppose."

Gwen smiled. "BO. Plain and simple."

Over the next few years I visited Gwen's place many times, mainly for the cats who had recurring bladder and skin problems. She never really got the flea thing completely under control although it certainly improved. I even met Ken vertically a couple of times. He was a quiet but personable type. He was very fond of Gwen, which apparently was a change from her previous husbands, about whom she'd told me a lot.

One afternoon, Gwen phoned me. She was sobbing. "It's Spot. He . . . he . . . can't get up. It's his b . . . b . . . back legs," she wept.

Ken took the phone. "I think he's busted one of his legs," he said. "He's been like it for a couple of days. Little fool fell down the stairs. Gwen didn't want to call you because she was frightened what your verdict might be. But I think you'd better come over. He doesn't look too flash."

"What if I come around after consulting tonight, about 7.30?"

"That'd be great, buddy. See you then."

That night I drove around with my new Scottish evening nurse, Eva. This, I thought, would be a good experience for her.

We walked into the building and immediately Cromagnon Man opened his creaky door.

Eva whispered in her strong Scottish accent, "Who's that?"

"That's the landlord," I whispered back. "He's a pig."

We knocked at Gwen's door and Ken opened.

"She's in there on the floor with him."

As we walked in I noticed Eva starting to blink

too. Her boyfriend smoked, but obviously nothing like Gwen and Ken. She stared at the chaos surrounding her. And there, among the ruins, was Gwen on the floor caressing Spot.

"Let him have a look, darl," Ken said, taking her by the arm.

She got up and with Eva's help I had a look at Spot's back legs. He'd broken his left hock badly. The bone was exposed and all the surrounding skin and muscle looked dry and lifeless. There was very little blood and the whole area was icy cold.

It didn't look promising, especially for a dog now seventeen years old.

"What do you reckon?" Ken asked.

"To be honest, I don't think we can do much for his leg."

"You mean you have to put him down."

"Well, aside from amputation, that's about all that's left."

With that Gwen lost it. Uncontrolled wailing. She hit the deck like a steel safe, throwing herself all over Spot and hugging and kissing him.

"Come on, darlin'," Ken said. "It's for the best. He's much too old for any operation."

"I know, I know," she cried.

Ken gently lifted her off the floor.

Eva and I then joined Spot on the floor and put him to sleep. He looked peaceful.

"Is that it? Is he gone?" Gwen asked.

"Yes, he's gone," I said.

The earlier episode of grief had only been a curtain-raiser before the main event. A tremor before the earthquake.

"Oh Spot!" she cried and dropped to the floor again, sobbing uncontrollably. I couldn't even see Spot. She had draped herself over his limp little body completely, feverishly kissing and patting his lifeless form.

We all stood there nonplussed. Normally, I was pretty good at consoling grieving pet owners. And Eva had shown herself to be quite adept at it too. But this was over the top. We didn't dare go near her.

"Come on, love," said Ken. "Let it go."

He reached down to lift her up but she wouldn't budge. She was shrieking with anguish and remorse.

"He's dead! He's dead! If only we'd called you earlier," she wailed.

"It wouldn't have made any difference," I assured her from a safe distance.

Ken tried to pull her off Spot again, this time a little more forcefully. But her grip was relentless. The more he pulled, the tighter she held.

"Come on, honey. This isn't helping anyone."

At one point he even put his foot on her hip for leverage as he pulled on her arm to try and get her to release her grip. I thought he was going to pull her arm out of its socket. Eva and I looked at each other trying not to laugh. If it hadn't been so sad it would have been funny.

Finally, enough was enough. Totally sapped of

energy and depleted of tears, Gwen slumped exhausted on her Spot. Ken, sensing it was safe to try again, bent down and was able to lift her off and take her over to sit on the bed.

"Thanks," he said to me. "We'll look after the little bloke from here."

Eva and I left without further comment and headed downstairs. Lo and behold, who should be standing at his sentry post again? Palaeolithic Man had probably heard the whole thing. He'd finished his pie, although some had remained around his mouth and on his singlet and shorts, and now he had a can of Coke in his hand.

I looked at him and smiled. "Cheers," I said, raising my hand with an imaginary glass. "Have a great evening."

He didn't say a thing, not a word. Just grunted and slunk back into his cave.

chapter 9

Tactical response

It was a cold wintry night and blowing an absolute gale outside. I was sitting in one of those trendy Paddington cafes having dinner with my friend Gary Brilley, who'd come down to Sydney for a few days on business from his property in Mudgee. We'd known each other for a number of years through his work as an insurance salesman and the friendship had grown from there.

On this particular evening we were discussing the prospects of a couple of slow racehorses we'd foolishly invested in. I was on call, and with my pager clipped to my pocket we spent the evening trying to talk above the music that was too loud, like it always is in those types of places.

We, or more accurately Gary, spoke about how our horses were going to make us millionaires. He was always the optimist and reckoned they were both "champions", but in the little I've had to do with racehorses and their owners it seemed like everyone had a future "champion". In fact, that word had become so overused that it seemed now to refer to any horse that managed to finish a race before the commercial break on TV.

Gary spoke enthusiastically and at length about the extensive family trees of these two thoroughbreds, with so many "out of this horse" and "by that horse", I figured our equine financial drains must have been the product of one of the greatest orgies ever known.

I must be fair though. They had won a few minor races in the country, which had at least covered some of their costs, but as soon as they raced in the city against any horse that didn't sit on the porch watching the sunset, they got flogged. We did run a creditable ninth at one city meeting, though, with our horse noticeably slowing at the finish. Then, after the race, we were bombarded with what I've discovered is another quaint racing tradition from jockeys and trainers after a resounding and humiliating loss — endless ridiculous excuses.

"If he'd had any luck at all in the race, he would have streeted them."

Of course, the only luck our horse could have hoped for was if the other horses hadn't shown up.

"He'll do a lot better than that when he gets a longer race. He was checked just as he was about to make his run."

And they would say all this with the unchallengeable conviction that racing people seem to have. I wanted to say: "It also would have helped if he could have run a bit," but this wasn't the time to let common sense get in the way.

At any rate, we'd settled into our coffee for the evening, with Gary puffing away on his Marlboros and telling me he could give up cigarettes any time he wanted, when my pager went off.

"Damn!" I grumbled. "Always at the wrong time."

"Just don't answer it." Gary always had simple solutions.

"No, I'd better. It might be something serious."

That's the thing about after-hours calls. Ninety per cent of them aren't emergencies, but you can't take the risk and ignore any of them.

I went over to the counter, explained my situation and asked to use the phone.

"Hello, it's Tony Sheldon from the veterinary hospital."

"G'day, it's Police Sergeant Grant," came the drawled reply. "We got this old lady whose little dog's just been mugged by a Rottweiler. She's in a bit of a state. Her little pooch's copped one hell of a hiding."

"Is he conscious?" I asked.

"Yeah, yeah, he's conscious. But one of his legs looks like it's hanging by a thread and there's a bit of blood dripping from his old fella," he continued laconically. "Don't reckon it looks too bloody good for him."

Sergeant Grant sounded like a bit of a stoic, an outback country type. I got the feeling no emergency was going to spur this man into overdrive. Except for his graphic description of the injuries, I had little to go on regarding the dog's general condition life-and-death-wise, but it sounded serious enough for me to get back to the hospital as quickly as possible.

"OK, Sergeant," I said. "I can meet you at the hospital in ten minutes. Keep the dog as warm as you can until I get there."

"Are you out somewhere, doc? I can hear music in the background."

"I was just having dinner." I had no idea where this line of questioning was going.

"Well, I don't want to be a bother and muck up your dinner. I can take care of things here."

"What do you mean, 'take care of things'?" I asked urgently. The situation was beginning to sound a little unstable.

"Well . . . it might be better to put him out of his misery," Sergeant Grant suggested, almost yawning.

"How? With a gun?"

"Yeah. We're allowed to do that if we think it's necessary."

"Where's the dog?"

"The old lady's got him on her lap. She's sitting on the kerb."

"And you're just going to shoot him there, in her lap?"

"Yeah, doc. It'll be quick."

I had no doubt it would be.

"But what if you miss?" I countered frantically.

"I never miss."

Stupid question. This was fast becoming a B-grade western. The slow-talking hulking deputy, bent at the knees, arms outstretched clasping tightly onto his gun about to blast this poor little dog as it sat trembling on a petrified old lady's lap. I had to act quickly.

"No, Sergeant. I really don't mind coming over. I've just finished dinner anyway. Who knows, maybe I'll be able to help him. Just tell the lady not to worry and that I'll be there shortly." I gave these instructions as calmly as I could, all things considered.

"OK, doc, but I hate to interrupt your dinner."

"Dinner's over," I repeated firmly.

I went back to the table, shaken by my encounter.

Gary was calmly sipping on his cappuccino, his cigarette in the cup-holding hand. "So, what was that all about?"

"You're not going to believe this. An old lady's little dog just got mauled by a Rottweiler, and the policeman on the phone offered to shoot him because he didn't want to disturb our dinner."

"What, shoot the Rottweiler?"

"No, the old lady's dog . . . while she's holding it."

Gary laughed. "You're kidding. Just blow the dog away at point-blank range? Is this bloke the full quid?"

"What do you think?"

"You'd better get out there quickly then. He sounds like he's looking for a reason."

Gary's imagination was as active as mine.

I sped out to the hospital as fast as I could.

Two policemen were waiting for me at the front door.

"You the doc?" asked the larger of the two. "I'm Sergeant Grant. I called you about the lady's dog."

He was exactly like I'd pictured him: tall, thick neck, heavy arms and legs and solid torso — the proverbial "brick outhouse" with a crew cut.

"Where is she?" I asked the man mountain.

"Across the road, sitting beside the patrol car. She's a bit shaken. Dog's a bloody mess. Don't think you'll be able to do much."

"So you've mentioned," I said sharply.

I was getting sick of being told how pointless my being there was. The old woman was sitting on the gutter, shivering and holding her dog. She somehow looked familiar.

"Would you kindly bring the woman and her dog in, please?" I was trying to speak as politely as I could, under the circumstances.

The other, much smaller, policeman walked over to where the woman sat, and helped her to her feet. He held onto her elbow as she carried her little Fox Terrier into the hospital.

I could see the extent of the damage to the left hind leg. The whole area around the groin was torn away. The little fellow, amazingly, wasn't complaining all that much; he just quietly buried his head in his mum's armpit and trembled a bit.

"What's his name?" I asked as I ushered her into the examination room.

"Timmy," she quivered. "I'm Mrs Kennedy. You desexed him a couple of years back." Then she paused for a moment and, looking down at his leg, said: "It's pretty bad, isn't it?"

"Well, Mrs Kennedy . . . it doesn't look all that good, but let's take a closer look."

I gently picked Timmy up and placed him on the examination table.

His injuries had miraculously not damaged any of the deeper blood vessels or nerves. There was certainly extensive skin and muscle damage, but his foot was still warm and he could withdraw it when I pinched his toes.

"I can't promise anything, Mrs Kennedy, but I think Timmy's got a chance."

"He does look pretty bad though, doesn't he, doc?" interjected Sergeant Grant, who'd snuck into the consulting room to watch. "Do you really think it's worth it?"

It was time to get rid of Dirty Harry. I didn't like his bedside manner. I also didn't like the way he always had his hand on his holster.

"I'll be OK now, Sergeant. I won't be needing you any more. Thanks a lot for helping out."

Once the police had left I explained to Mrs Kennedy that her dog's operation was going to be fairly difficult. There would be a long recovery period and there could be complications.

She was holding Timmy in her lap again. "You gotta give him a go though, don't you. He was my husband's best little mate, before he died last year," she said, first looking at Timmy and then to me. "Yes, let's give him a go. Jack would have wanted that."

I operated on Timmy that night and everything went well.

When Mrs Kennedy came in the next morning Timmy was still very sore and sorry, but he looked up and gave a token tail wag and an attempt at a bark. Mrs Kennedy was thrilled.

She checked on him each day and brought him small parcels of his favourite food. We were all very pleased and quite honestly surprised with the speed of his progress.

After a week in hospital Timmy was starting to be able to bear weight on his leg, and there was no sign of infection. It was time for him to go home.

He seemed to sense that Mrs Kennedy's next visit wasn't going to be a normal one. When she opened the cage door he jumped into her arms.

"OK, let's go home now," he seemed to say. "I'm better."

There was extravagant licking and kissing, a whole feast of bacterial exchange. This continued out the door, up the street and probably for some time at home too.

A week later Timmy came back for his suture removal. He had barely a limp, and the wound looked greatly improved.

"I'm so thankful for what you did," Mrs Kennedy effused. "It was such an awful accident."

A couple of months after the Timmy incident I was walking back from the newsagent's when I saw across the road the figure of a hulking policeman with a crew cut and those mirrored sunglasses. He was standing there, with his massive arms folded, talking to some terrified young kid about a defect or something on his car.

Sergeant Grant noticed me.

"Hey, doc!" he called out, and crossed the road to meet me. "Remember me? I helped you with that poor little dog a while back. You remember, the one that copped a shellacking from that Rotty."

People often have very strange interpretations of what constitutes help.

"Yes. I remember you were there."

"Didn't make it, did he?" he said almost triumphantly. "I knew you were wasting your time."

"Actually, he went pretty well."

"Really?" he said, and then with a chuckle: "Lucky I didn't shoot him then."

"Yeah, lucky."

chapter 10

Rainy days and Mondays

It was one of those awful wet days. One of those days when you watch the sky get blacker by the minute. And then the heavens open up and the roads become awash within seconds. It was one of those days if, for some stupid reason, you have to venture outside you are soaked to the skin immediately. Every single drop of rain is huge.

I hate those days. They are dirty days. The waiting room floor is slippery and grubby. People come in wet and filthy. It's not their fault. It is just that all the dirt and leaves from the street seem to gravitate towards and then stick to the soles of their shoes and then deposit themselves on the floor. We used to have a doormat for that reason but it kept getting stolen, and half the people were in such a rush to get in out of the rain that they never used it anyway. So we stopped buying them. Also at these times — for a reason I've never been able to fathom — dogs are more likely to urinate on the furniture when they come in. God, I hate those days.

It is also not a good time to upset the nurses. You would be well advised to tread gently around them. Their gallant efforts to keep a clean surgery are pretty much wasted. No sooner have they mopped the floor than someone will walk in, saturated with his or her full quota of dirt and leaves. And this person will invariably have a dog that shakes itself dry and lifts its leg. On those days cats are more belligerent too. Either being taken from the warmth of their homes, or getting wet in transit, seems to get them more agitated than usual.

It was on such a day I was called out to visit Mrs Granger.

"Hello, Mr Sheldon," came her frail voice, "Could you come out and have a look at my cat, Sylvester? He's very poorly."

I looked out the window at the monsoon. I was obviously being punished for something.

"What seems to be the problem?"

"Oh, he's sneezing and coughing all the time, and he doesn't want to eat at all. And his eyes, they're so red and they've got all this yellow stuff coming out of them."

"It sounds like he's got the 'flu, Mrs Granger. I can pop out and have a look him this afternoon. Is that convenient for you?"

I was hoping she'd say that tomorrow would be

just as good, what with the weather being as bad as it was.

"Yes, that would be wonderful," she said. "I'll be in all day with this terrible weather."

Good for some.

There was a pause, and then she added: "By the way, Mr Sheldon, I'm on the ground floor, but that's actually one floor down on the elevator."

I wasn't looking forward to this visit. I didn't have an umbrella, at least not one that would have been any good in this deluge. I was going to get drenched, absolutely drowned-rat drenched. The sooner I came to terms with that the better.

I'd finished the day's surgery by about mid afternoon and prepared what I'd need for Sylvester. As I was about to leave, all I could think about was getting to my car quickly. I picked up the house-call bag and ran. The car was only about four metres away in the driveway. I reached the driver's side door and felt for the keys in my pocket. They weren't there. I felt in the other pocket. They weren't there either. I was getting absolutely soaked. I felt in both pockets again. I ran back inside and there was Martina, waiting at the door, dangling the keys in her hand.

"Looking for these?"

I snatched them and ran back out to the car. I said nothing.

I arrived at the large, grey block of flats where Mrs Granger lived. It was one of several dull twelve-storey council blocks, made even duller by the dark skies.

There was a long footpath leading from the road to the building's entrance. I picked up a towel from the back seat of the car, draped it over my head, grabbed my bag, and ran like hell.

Following Mrs Granger's instructions I took the elevator down to the ground floor. It clunked to an abrupt halt and the door opened. My jaw dropped. The whole ground floor was under fifteen centimetres of water. There were two steps leading up to the door of each apartment, which ultimately saved the occupants from being completely flooded too.

Mrs Granger was in number seven, four doors down. The distance between units was too far to jump from one stair to the next. I was left with only one option — I'd have to take off my shoes and socks and wade across. So I sat on the floor in the lift, keeping the door open with one foot while I took the shoe and sock off the other, and then changed feet to repeat the process. With shoes and socks in one hand, medical bag in the other, and trousers rolled up to the knees, I set off through the rising tide for apartment number seven.

Standing on the doorstep fully laden I pressed the buzzer with the only appendage available, my nose. Mrs Granger had told me it would take a little time for her to answer, as she had a disability.

A minute or so later came a frail voice: "Who is it?"

"It's Tony Sheldon . . . the vet."

The door opened and there stood a tiny old woman supporting herself with an ornate walking stick. The handpiece was carved in the shape of a duck's head. Mrs Granger had been expecting me and so had dressed up a bit: a neat blue dress, a string of pearls, and her silver hair tied neatly in a bun. My guess was that her social calendar was probably a bit thin and that she enjoyed having a visitor, even if it was just the vet coming to look at Sylvester.

"Come in, Mr Sheldon, come in. It's so good of you to come."

I was bewildered. She didn't appear to notice that I was standing there like a bedraggled orphan dripping on her carpet. At least she didn't make mention of it. As I followed her into the living room her disability became evident. She had one stiff leg, her right, and had to move it in an arc as she walked.

"There's Sylvester, on the chair. He's been so ill."

Sylvester was a scrawny old male tabby. He had a yellow discharge from his nose and eyes, and sounded blocked up even from a distance.

I looked at him and he stared unblinkingly back at me. I put my shoes and socks on the floor and, as I took one step towards him, he jumped off the chair and ran straight into the bedroom and under the bed.

This visit was going to take longer than I'd planned.

"Oh dear. I'm so sorry. I knew I should have kept that door shut."

That would have been helpful.

I followed Sylvester into the bedroom. Mrs Granger had one of those ensemble beds on castors.

The ten or twelve centimetres between the bed base and the carpet were just enough to fit a cat comfortably.

I lay down on my stomach to see under the bed.

Sylvester was in the middle — dead centre. I tried to reach him with my hand but didn't come close.

"Come on, Sylvester, I won't hurt you," I pleaded.

He knew that wasn't true. Cats know everything.

To get closer I squeezed my head sideways under the sagging mattress. I kept pushing until my head was stuck, my face contorted and pressed firmly against the carpet. Sylvester just stared at me. He made no attempt to move. He knew I couldn't reach him. Cats have some internal radar system that tells them exactly where under a piece of furniture they are unreachable from any point.

My attempts to capture him were failing miserably. It occurred to me how ridiculous this must look. A grown man, soaking wet, lying stomach down on the floor, his face squashed and disfigured under a bed, pleading to a cat who was surely reassessing which of the two was lower on the food chain.

Discouraged but not beaten, I pulled my head out — giving my face carpet burn in the process — and considered my options. Mrs Granger was now also in the bedroom standing next to her dresser. I had an idea.

"Mrs Granger, would I be able to borrow your walking stick for a moment? I might be able to get Sylvester out with that."

I thought I might be able to drag him out like they used to do with bad vaudeville acts. I figured I could hook him with the duck's beak.

"Oh yes, Mr Sheldon. What a good idea."

She handed me her stick and held onto her bedside table for support.

I resumed my position of dignity on the floor and exposed the new weapon to my now complacent adversary. As I edged the stick around him he showed the first signs of concern. That in itself was a moral victory. I pulled the stick toward me and with it Sylvester. The lowness of the bed now worked against him, as he couldn't jump back over the stick. Soon he was within hand's reach. I grabbed his scruff and managed to pull him out.

"You've got him, Mr Sheldon, you've got him! How wonderful." Mrs Granger clapped her hands together with joy, and in her overzealous display started to lose her balance. As she started to sag downward she quickly grabbed hold of the bedside table again. With my free hand I hastily passed back her stick, and she grabbed it as urgently as if it were a lifebuoy and sat down on the chair on the other side of the table. It had been quite a shock for her and it took some minutes before she was able to recover her poise.

"Good gracious." Her voice was trembling. "I really must be a little more careful."

Surprisingly, throughout all of this calamity, I managed to maintain my grip on Sylvester's scruff. He didn't hiss or growl. By and large he accepted his capture quite well. I sat down on the bed and proceeded to examine him.

The diagnosis wasn't difficult. The description over the phone had been enough. With the wet weather he'd caught a bad dose of the 'flu and was feverish. I put him on a course of antibiotics which usually settled these things in a few days. Mrs Granger assured me she would have no trouble giving Sylvester his tablets, as she had managed it many times before.

There was no point in putting my shoes back on at this stage, as I was going to have to wade back to the lift, so I left as I had come in.

It was still pouring outside but there was no reason to rush. I was still wet, and dirty and tired. I stomped through every puddle on the footpath, like a kid, making sure I didn't miss any until reaching the car.

I arrived back at the hospital in the same damp state I had been at Mrs Granger's doorstep.

Martina just looked at me dripping everywhere. "You'd better not pee on the furniture," she said.

chapter 11

Fat chance

"Hello? Is that Dr Sheldon?" came a concerned voice with a heavy German accent. "Can you come and have a look at my Robbie?"

So started my colourful association with Mr and Mrs Heinricht.

Mrs Heinricht was German and seventy something — Mr Heinricht was Russian and his age was anyone's guess — and had one of those heavily lined but kindly faces that somehow mirror a life that's had more than its fair share of hardship and tragedy. She was tallish and bespectacled and, like many elderly European women, she maintained a pride in her appearance, always being well groomed on the occasions I visited her home.

Mr Heinricht — or "Villie" as his wife called him — was a very different kettle of fish. A thin, frail, balding man, Willie liked a drink. Actually, Willie liked to drink very much more than any liver should be asked to accommodate. That's probably why his age was so hard to evaluate. His long battle with the bottle had left him physically ravaged.

I remember the first visit well. I knocked at the door of their tiny, single-storey, inner-city terrace. Out the front there was no little garden, not even a pot plant. It was all concrete and painted yellow.

Mrs Heinricht answered my knock. "Hello, doctor. I'm so glad to see you. My Robbie's very sick."

As I walked in, I was startled by a slurred roar from my left. *"Hello, doctor!"* There was Willie, lying on his back on a bed under the window, his head propped up on a pillow, his shirt open and his fly completely undone. He was either unaware or was just past caring.

"Hello, doctor!" he roared again, proudly holding up a bottle of beer. "You've come to see my Robbie."

As I was to discover, the Heinrichts had first met in Australia in the late thirties, having escaped the Nazi invasion of Europe, as my own parents had done. Every time I came to see their three dogs, Willie would proudly and incessantly relate his daring escape across Russia. Obviously Willie had chosen to deal with his painful memories differently from his wife. He would drown them.

As I was escorted across the living room I was enthusiastically greeted by a Dachshund and a Kelpie: Maxie and Klaus. They were both fat and the reason lay at various points throughout the house.

There were huge bowls of food left for them all day, so they could eat whenever and as much as they desired.

"Get down, Max! Klaus!" Mrs Heinricht pleaded as they jumped all over me. "I'm sorry, doctor."

The adjoining room was the kitchen, cluttered with cutlery and plates piled high in the sink and on the sideboards. And in one corner of the kitchen lay Robbie. He was a grossly overweight Golden Labrador-cross, the largest of the three dogs by far. He was lying on his side, panting furiously, and appeared to be in terrible distress.

"That's my poor Robbie," said Mrs Heinricht. "He's been like that for three days . . . and vomiting all the time. I wanted to call you earlier, but I thought he would get better."

I felt Robbie's abdomen. It was rock hard, and he would moan if I put any sort of pressure on it at all. He was running a fever of 41 degrees Celsius and was very dehydrated because of all the vomiting. His excessive weight was a problem I often saw in pets living with old, inactive people whose prime means of bestowing their love and affection was through food.

"What do you feed him?" I asked, knowing full well what the answer would be.

"He eats everything we eat," Mrs Heinricht replied hesitantly. "Is that not good?"

Usually "everything we eat" means leftovers such as the fat trimmed off the chops or the dripping from the evening roast. And there were also those massive bowls of food left all over the house during the day. It was a diet for disaster.

"Mrs Heinricht," I said firmly, "you are feeding Robbie and the others way too much. I think his pancreas has become very inflamed. That's why he's so sick."

Mrs Heinricht nodded, but I could tell she had no idea what I was talking about. I would try to explain his impending treatment more simply. "I'm going to have to ——"

"Doctor! How's my Robbie?" Willie had managed to drag himself off the bed to see what was happening. He was swaying and smiling one of those "the lights are on but nobody's home" type smiles.

"Be quiet, Villie. The doctor is trying to tell me about Robbie."

That instruction cruised harmlessly over his hazy head.

"So, doctor, how are you?" came Willie again, smiling blankly from his own little inebriated netherworld. (I was to discover that Willie often joined in the proceedings with things totally unrelated to what was going on.)

"I'm fine, but Robbie's not too good," I replied, trying to return attention to the matter at hand.

"I remember when I was sick like Robbie, when I was escaping from those bloody Nazis."

"Villie! Be quiet!" Mrs Heinricht looked skyward in exasperation.

Mrs Heinricht, while generally tolerant, would

sometimes lose her patience with him, much like a mother berating her ever-annoying child.

I began again. "I'm going to have to take Robbie to hospital with me. He is really very unwell. I hope we'll be able to get him through all of this."

With that I picked up the four-legged medicine ball, marginally avoided a hernia, and headed back through the house on my way to the car. I passed Willie, who was now back sitting on the edge of the bed, drinking again, a little dejected after the last dressing-down from his wife.

"You look after my Robbie," he pleaded, still hampered by his intoxication.

I put Robbie on the back seat of the car and drove back to the hospital, to the constant sounds of his groaning.

It was touch and go. We had Robbie on a drip for five days until he turned the corner. I phoned Mrs Heinricht with the news. She was thrilled and, I felt, a little surprised that he was coming home at all.

I arrived back at the house and knocked on the door. Robbie stood by my side, wagging his entire body in anticipation. Mrs Heinricht answered the door, and Robbie, handicapped by his still not insignificant weight, made valiant if unsuccessful attempts to jump for joy.

Mrs Heinricht put her finger to her lips. "Shh, shh, Villie's asleep and it's been so peaceful. Come on through to the kitchen."

We tiptoed through the living room and stood in

the kitchen whispering. I took pains to explain that we had been lucky to pull Robbie through and that it was absolutely vital that she cut down his food, as we may not be so lucky next time.

She said she understood but, judging by her and Robbie's mutual happiness at being reunited, I knew food was soon to change hands. I only hoped it would be a moderate portion, although I knew deep down that after an initial period of token restraint, Robbie would again be dining at the Ritz.

As we walked back into the living room where Willie slept, she looked at him and said with some despair: "I really don't know why I married him. He's been such a burden, and at my age . . ." There was no malice in her words. She just seemed tired.

"The only man I ever really loved was my first husband," she continued, seemingly happy to have someone other than Willie to talk to.

I felt a personal confidence coming on.

"What happened to him?" I asked, and immediately sensed I shouldn't have. I had a feeling the answer was not going to be simple and would probably be embarrassing.

"He had many affairs."

I was beginning to feel uncomfortable. I just knew she was going to elaborate.

"He said I made love like a peasant."

My instincts were correct. Some very graphic and intimate secrets were about to be divulged. I was starting to get anxious. "Oh," I said meekly, as though responding to some mundane question about the weather.

I wasn't actually aware peasants made love differently to other women, but I also didn't want an explanation of what that difference was. So I began to frantically organise Robbie's medicine, in the hope of ending the prospect of any expansion of the topic. After all, her first marriage must have ended at least fifty years ago, surely time enough to get over it. But then as I looked across at her drunken little Bolshevik asleep on the bed I could understand her need to resurrect the past. But really, I was only the vet. My first and last foray into sexual therapy had ended many years ago, with Norbert, the Great Dane.

Sensing that I was uneasy with details of her love life, Mrs Heinricht smiled and said: "You've done such a good job with my Robbie. How much do I owe you?"

Because they were on a pension, and because the bill was six hundred and twenty dollars, I began by saying I would be happy if they paid it in instalments. But Mrs Heinricht wouldn't hear of it. Instead, this elderly, elegant woman nonchalantly lifted her dress high, exposing a thigh that must have once looked better. There was a thick, frilly black garter belt strapped around it.

I was becoming very uncomfortable. The tightness in my chest returned. Was this going to become really weird? Was she now, some five decades later, going to try and disprove the peasant theory? If she tried to kiss or touch me I'd pass out, for sure. Or was this just a decorative tourniquet to help alleviate the bleeding condition she suffered from and which she had earlier mentioned. And if the latter was the case, why was it important for me to see it?

My worries, however, were unfounded. She simply reached down and from her garter extracted a bundle of notes, and paid the bill in full. I've never been so relieved.

"Thank you again, Dr Sheldon," she said. "You've made us very happy."

As I was leaving, Robbie waddled over to his master, who was out cold on the bed, and licked his face. Willie half woke and patted the wagging torso. "Robbie, you're back."

chapter 12

Old troupers

I hadn't seen Doc Davies since his last cat, Raaf, died of old age a few years back. He was twenty-eight when he went. Or so Doc told me.

"Are you sure he's twenty-eight?" I'd asked at the time. People tended to exaggerate the age of their elderly animals. It seems their merit as an owner was directly proportional to how long their pet lived.

"Well," Doc explained, looking up to collect his thoughts. "We buried Tornado Ted twenty-six years ago. He was my mate in the 85th Airborne. I remember that because it was also my fortieth birthday that day. So we had a party and a wake all on the same night. We had them at different pubs though. Out of respect. Teddy got the big C. Some sort of chemical or something they used in the war. Anyway, I had Raaf then and he was young but fully grown, so he's got to be at least twenty-seven."

"Hello, Tony," now came a voice I couldn't properly place. "It's Doc Davies. Davies of Dampier Street."

He always introduced himself on the phone that way. But this time he sounded much frailer than I remembered.

"Can you come over this afternoon and have a look at my cat Dunkirk?" he went on. "His skin is really bad. He's so itchy, chewing and licking all the time. I've been breaking off the scabs but they keep coming back."

That wasn't a recognised treatment for dermatitis.

This was only the second time, in all the years I'd seen his animals, that he'd ever asked for a house call, so that made me wonder a bit. Maybe he'd just pranged his car like the first time.

"And do you think you'd be able to come before two? I've got a few crook mates in hospitals and nursing homes I've got to visit later on."

He didn't live far away, so I slotted him in between operations and headed out around midday.

I soon arrived at the tiny lime-green inner-city terrace nestled toward the end of the street. The small front porch was all concrete, but nature was busy forcing its way through the cracks.

An old, unshaven man answered the door still in dressing gown and slippers. For him, morning had come and gone pretty much unnoticed. He made a futile attempt to get his unkempt hair into some semblance of order as he welcomed me in.

"G'day, Tony. Thanks for fitting me in. Dunkirk's over here."

This wasn't the Doc Davies I remembered. He'd aged fifteen years in the last three. And inside the place was a mess, cluttered with old books, old vaudeville posters and even older dust. Unswept leaves had blown in from outside and the odd used plastic wrapper lay undisturbed on the floor. A crackling old black and white television was on and it was ghosting badly. There was hardly room to walk. It all had the dank smell of a stagnant life. I instinctively brushed a cobweb off a broken chest of drawers that sat awkwardly on a coffee table pushed up against a wall.

It was sad to see because Doc had been such a vibrant performer all his life. One of the real characters. He did the clubs as a one-man band. The only other time I'd been to see him at his home he gave me a musical recital, although "musical" was stretching the truth some. Those one-man band catastrophes always looked to me like some poor coot trapped in a disorganised scaffolding of musical instruments flailing frantically to get out. It was just purposeless loud noise. Like mob violence. And everything was always drowned out by the clash of those mandatory huge cymbals. His rendition that day of "We'll Meet Again" would not have inspired the war effort. Even Vera Lynn would have been hard pressed to recognise it.

Now as I followed him through the house I started

to get itchy around the ankles. This skin problem was going to be easy to diagnose.

Dunkirk was sitting on top of an old picture of Roy Rene that looked like it was never going to be hung. He was a three-year-old Burmese who spent all his time obsessively grooming. I parted the fur along his back and watched as the first battalion of fleas hastily made a tactical retreat. They'd obviously gone to summon reinforcements. I continued my examination up the neck to the head. There were hundreds of them, running across the bridge of his nose and crawling into his ears. The skin all over his body was covered with inflamed crusts.

"Have you seen all these fleas?" I asked Doc.

"Is that what it is?" he replied. "Well, who would have thought?"

Who would have thought? An entire Panzer Division was about to walk away with his cat and he couldn't see it?

"Look here," I said, again parting the fur on Dunkirk's back. "There's millions of them."

"I suppose I should have noticed," he lamented, "but I'm going blind. Have been for the past year. See that photo of me on the shelf over there?"

He pointed to a glossy enlargement sitting next to an old framed copy of the original manuscript of Banjo Paterson's "Waltzing Matilda". In the photo Doc was in full cowboy get-up — gun, holster, leather chaps, ten-gallon hat, the whole shebang. And in his hand he was holding a violin and bow.

"I was going to play my fiddle as Cowboy Bob. Had the gigs all lined up."

I never knew he played the violin, or fiddle as he called it. I thought he only played that flesh-eating mass of steel that now sat rusting in the corner of the living room.

"But about a year ago the doctor told me I had macula degeneration and that I'd eventually be completely blind. I can play the fiddle with my eyes closed but the organisers were worried I'd fall off the edge of the stage," he added with a resigned chuckle.

I looked around at the fading furniture and the mountains of decaying memorabilia lying randomly throughout. So this is what lost hope looks like?

"So how are you coping?" I asked, as if his surroundings weren't evidence enough.

"Oh, pretty good, Tone. I just wish I could look after Dunkirk a bit better."

"Do you think you'd be able to wash him?" I ventured. "Because he's going to need a flea bath before we do anything else."

"Oh dear! I'd never be able to do that. He can be a bit contrary at times. You know what cats are like."

I didn't really expect he'd be able to. It's hard enough for someone who can see what they're doing.

"I'll tell you what," I offered. "I'm off on Saturday. I'll pop over and give you a hand."

"Would you? I'd be so thankful."

I gave Dunkirk an injection to stop the itch and drove back to the surgery.

That night I lay in bed and thought about Doc and old age. The only things left in his life were Dunkirk, his infirm old war mates and his macula degeneration. He appeared to derive a certain pride in that disease with its fancy medical name. It seemed, I suppose, that if you were going to go blind it may as well be with something that sounded exotic. To me "macula degeneration" sounded like Mary's part in the birth of Jesus. All I knew about it was that dogs and cats didn't get it.

And poor Dunkirk. He was an absolute mess. He'd become a McDonald's for fleas and the franchise was killing him.

Saturday morning and I arrived for the Big Wash. Doc was out of his dressing gown and ready for business. Our forthcoming task had given his adrenaline a much-needed boost.

When I walked back into the house it was like stepping out of the real world and back into a life that existed independently of it.

"So, you ready for this?" I asked.

"Ready as I'll ever be," he said, rubbing his hands together. "Not too sure about Dunkirk though. He must have sensed something. He's up on top of the cupboard over there, the one sitting on the couch."

That structure didn't look overly stable. Memories of Sylvester flooded back.

Dunkirk had planted his flag on the highest point inside the house. He looked down at base camp and assessed his situation. He must have thought to himself, "Now that Doc has that macula thing, he's got no likelihood of reaching me up here. And that young bloke who was messing with me the other day, he's got Buckley's of making this sort of a climb. I'm safe."

"Anything that's in your way, just push it to the side," Doc instructed.

I figured there wouldn't be a problem in disturbing the order of things.

So away went the framed poster of the Marx Brothers and the metal vice (God knows what that was doing in the living room). I shifted a huge pile of old books, which disturbed a pile of resting dust.

Coughing and rubbing the dust from my eyes I climbed onto the couch and pulled out one of the drawers of the cupboard to use as a step.

"Can you hold onto the cupboard while I climb up?" I asked Doc.

"OK, Tone. There, it's steady now."

I climbed up the tower which, despite Doc's assurances, was anything but steady. Fortunately it was at least in part leaning against the wall, which afforded some sense of security, however tenuous. Doc had his arms wrapped around the cupboard like a fond memory.

When I finally scaled my Everest and reached Dunkirk he was surprisingly reconciled to his capture. I had expected some resistance, a hiss, a claw, at the very least a handshake on a climb well done. But the contemptuous look on his face seemed to say, "So what? You climbed up a stupid cupboard. I was coming down anyway."

Cats don't appreciate courage.

I grabbed him by the scruff with one hand and used the other to climb down.

"Where do you want to do this?" I asked Doc.

"The bath's as good a place as any. I let in a bit of warm water just before you came."

Once we had Dunkirk in the bath we started to lather him up. The water soon turned red as the flea dirt dissolved in it.

"See how red the water is?" I said to Doc. "That's because of all the flea dirt."

"Yes, I can see that."

His less than convincing tone suggested he probably couldn't.

"So who are you visiting this afternoon?" I asked to pass the time as we sent Dunkirk disappearing in a mass of suds.

"I've got to see old Mike. They used to call him Maniac Mike when he was a tail gunner with me in the war. God he was fearless. You wouldn't believe it to see him now. Poor bloke had a stroke. Now his left side's about as good as my eyes. His arm just hangs there."

Dunkirk looked at us both disdainfully. He'd obviously decided that to struggle would only prolong the indignity. He just wished we'd shut up and get on with it.

"I could easily shred Doc," he must have thought

as he stood soaking wet. "But he's my soulmate. We go back a way."

Then he looked squarely at me. "But I should give the young bloke a jolt just so he doesn't think he's had it all his own way."

We washed and rewashed Dunkirk and poured a flea rinse over him. Then we lifted him onto the dresser by the bath and towelled him dry. He looked much better, many of the scabs having disappeared following the injection I'd given him earlier. Doc patted him on the head as I vigorously rubbed him down.

When we'd finished he gladly jumped off the dresser and rushed straight to the food bowl.

I explained to Doc that this was only the beginning. He still had to flea bomb the house and give Dunkirk medicine once a month so any fleas he may pick up outside couldn't breed.

"Yeah, I can do that," he said. Then he walked into his bedroom and came out with his chequebook.

"I'll just sign this and you can fill it in for how much I owe you."

It occurred to me how easy it must be for conmen to take advantage of such people.

He put the cheque on a little round table in the lounge room.

"This is where I sign, right?" he asked as he slowly lowered his hand to the paper.

He was just about to sign an RSL coaster sitting below the cheque. He obviously hadn't seen the water turn red. I gently pushed the cheque down to where his hand looked like it was going and said: "Yes, that's right."

Dunkirk was now sitting on the broken chest of drawers I'd passed as I came in. As I walked by to leave, he lashed out with a lightning-fast right cross, drawing blood from my forearm.

"That's just so you know who really won here," he smirked.

chapter 13

Glasnost in Surry Hills

I heard an earsplitting bang on the front glass doors of the surgery.

"My God! What was that?" I called out to Martina, who was sitting at the reception desk.

"Mrs Ivanof. She's just walked into the front door again."

I glanced around the corner to see Svetlana Ivanof still shaking her head, walking in on the arm of elderly Boris Ivanof. They were old-world Russian and looked misplaced in the hurly-burly of the big city.

It was a cold morning and he was wearing what was obviously a hand-knitted beanie over his almost totally bald head. Faded leather braces held up a pair of ancient baggy trousers, and tucked into them was a grey sweater — a much-cherished sweater, judging by the degree of wear it showed.

Mrs Ivanof had adjusted to the twentieth century a little better. She wore a colourful modern dress, and her shoes had slightly raised heels. She also wore the thickest glasses I'd ever seen — the lenses must have been two centimetres thick. It was difficult to look at her face-on because those lenses magnified her eyes, making her look like a fish. And they didn't work. They didn't work at all. As far as I could tell she was still as blind as a bat.

In her free arm she held her fourteen-year-old Chihuahua, Pepe. Everyone seemed to call their Chihuahuas Pepe, or sometimes Pancho.

I directed them into the consulting room, carefully steering Mrs Ivanof safely through the door, and motioned for them to place Pepe on the examination table.

"No piss. No piss." Mr Ivanof pointed to his own crotch to clarify the point.

They spoke very little English. We always did the best we could with sign language. Fortunately, this problem was fairly straightforward.

I felt Pepe's abdomen. His bladder was rock hard and the size of a small orange. I applied gentle pressure which caused him severe pain and he was still unable to urinate. The bladder was obstructed, and that was an emergency. I was sure Pepe had bladder stones. The immediate dilemma was trying to explain that to the Ivanofs.

"Stones. Stones in bladder," I said, depicting a stone by indicating a small imaginary object between my index finger and thumb and then also ridiculously pointing to my crotch. I repeated this gesture over and over a number of times, but I don't think they grasped the stone concept. They kept nodding as though they understood, but I think they just thought I was telling them Pepe had a small penis.

Maybe they would understand X-rays. That was pretty universal and it was the only way to positively diagnose the condition anyway.

"We X-ray Pepe. X-ray Pepe," I suggested.

I don't know why we always repeat ourselves when trying to explain something to people who don't speak our own language. If they didn't understand it the first time, why would they the second?

But, fortunately, in this case they understood X-ray after I pointed to one, and nodded their approval for me to go ahead with it.

"Please sit. Please sit," I gestured with my hand as they walked back into the waiting room.

I then took Pepe and started to walk to Radiology. I was half way there when my progress was slowed by a strange tugging on my belt. I thought I must have caught it on something, but when I looked around there was old Mr Ivanof, who'd hooked his index finger into my belt and was following me.

"No, no, please sit. Only one minute. One minute." I unhooked his finger, and escorted him back to sit with his wife. I gestured gently with my free hand for them to sit and stay while I took the X-rays.

Pepe was co-operative, needing no sedation, and

soon Martina and I had the radiographs. His bladder was full of stones, one of which was stuck half way down the penis. That was the problem.

I asked the Ivanofs back into the consulting room so I could show them the pictures. Mrs Ivanof carelessly walked ahead of her husband and her shoulder clipped the door as she walked in. How was she going to see an X-ray?

I attached the X-ray to the viewer on the wall and pointed out the stones to Mr Ivanof. I was greeted with a nod and a blank stare.

"See? Stones in bladder," I said, pointing to them. Then, with my finger, I traced the path of the one that was stuck, showing him how it came to be lodged where it was.

"This one stuck here. Stuck here. No piss." I was repeating myself again and getting absolutely nowhere, and I couldn't believe I'd resorted to that last description.

Mr Ivanof gave a confused shrug of the shoulders. Mrs Ivanof wasn't even looking at the right wall.

"See here, stuck. This one stuck," I said, as I pointed to the stone and then to my own crotch again. I even pointed to Mr Ivanof's crotch. This was going badly.

It was becoming unbelievably frustrating that I wasn't getting through to them. I could feel my jaw clenching and hear my voice rising an octave.

I was trying valiantly to stay calm, despite wanting to bang my head hard against the wall and scream:

"It's simple! Why can't you understand me?"

"My daughter. You call," Mrs Ivanof suggested, handing me a business card.

It was like sighting land after floating aimlessly at sea for days.

"Hello, can I speak to Katrina Ivanof?"

"Speaking," came the reply, devoid of any accent. It was like music to my ears. My blood pressure dropped and I regained my equilibrium.

"It's Tony Sheldon from the vet hospital. I've got your parents here with Pepe and I'm having a little trouble explaining his problem."

"What's the matter with him?"

"He's got bladder stones and they need to be removed. Can you explain it to them?"

I passed the phone to Mrs Ivanof and waited for the outcome of several minutes of emotive Russian.

She gave the phone back.

"Is that an operation?" Katrina asked.

"Yes it is."

"They don't want an operation. They think he's too old."

"Well, he's not going to get much older if we don't."

"Let me talk to my mother again."

I passed the phone over to Mrs Ivanof and waited. After several minutes she gave the phone back to me.

"What's the alternative, she wants to know," said Katrina.

"Well, we can try to flush the blocked stone back

into the bladder with the others and then try to dissolve them over time, medically."

"Give me my mother again."

I felt like a switchboard operator. More Russian dialogue followed and Mrs Ivanof gave me the phone again.

"She wants to try that," Katrina relayed.

"OK, but the very likely risk is that before they finally dissolve one could get stuck again."

"Let me talk to my mother again."

My land-sighting had been a mirage. Still more colourful Russian. Mr Ivanof, through this whole drama, stood passively beside his wife with his hands behind his back.

Katrina spoke to me again. "OK, do the surgery."

"Good," I said quickly, before they could change their mind. "Call me this evening at five and I'll let you know how everything went."

I hung up the phone quickly, to avoid any second thoughts.

Having agreed on our plan of action I took Pepe from the Ivanofs, headed off with him into the kennel area and gave him his pre-med.

Thirty minutes later Martina came to me. "They're still out in the waiting room."

I walked out and there they were, both sitting there like lost children, with their hands in their laps, looking blankly ahead.

"You can go home now," I said. "Pepe is OK. Katrina will call me later."

They smiled and Mr Ivanof took his wife's arm and escorted her out.

Pepe's surgery went well. We managed to flush the stone back into the bladder and take it out along with all the others.

At five on the dot the phone rang. "Hello, it's Katrina Ivanof. How's Pepe?"

"He's fine. He got through the surgery well. We managed to remove all the stones and he should be able to go home tomorrow."

"That's wonderful. My parents were so worried."

Then, even though it was none of my business, I ventured: "By the way, have you seen your mother lately? I don't think her glasses are working very well."

"I know," Katrina sighed. "But she's much worse without them."

I couldn't see how that was possible.

This had been a tiring day. The Ivanof affair had left me drained. Pepe had recovered well from his operation and was sleeping comfortably. Martina, who lived above the hospital, could keep a check on him and phone me if anything went wrong during the night.

I drove home and sank mindlessly in front of the television. I was hungry but didn't have the energy to cook, so I rang a home-delivery service and ordered some Mexican. It arrived about forty minutes later and after polishing it off in ten minutes I dragged myself off to sleep. Getting into a warm bed when you're dead tired is one of the purest pleasures in life.

Soon I was fast asleep, deeply and blissfully cut off from the pressures of the day.

Then, like a jackhammer, the phone rang, brutally shaking my slumber. I looked at the clock, squinting in order to focus. It was after eleven. Who could possibly . . . ?

"Hi, Tone. It's Rob."

Rob was one of my closest friends. He was a vet too and had a practice a fair way out of Sydney.

"What's up?" I asked feebly. "It's nearly midnight."

"This guy's dog just jumped off the Harbour Bridge. He's pretty bad. I told the guy to take him straight around to your hospital."

"Yeah, right." I hung up the phone. This was obviously a poor joke.

The phone rang immediately again.

"Don't hang up. It's true."

"So how'd they fish him out of the water? He'd have to be dead."

"He didn't jump in the water, idiot. He was chasing pigeons above the Argyle Cut and jumped off that. I was doing a sculpture course down here at The Rocks and heard this awful thud outside. Everyone ran out."

"What sort of dog is it?" I asked.

"It's a Doberman. The guy will probably be there in about fifteen."

"Thanks a lot."

I dragged myself out of bed, put on my tracksuit and fumbled for my keys. I was on automatic pilot as I drove to the surgery. As I headed around the back I saw that people were already waiting at the front.

I opened up and they carried Tyson in and put him on the floor next to the examination table. We were going through a period where almost everyone with a Doberman, Rottweiler or a Bull Terrier was calling them Tyson or Rocky.

I was surprised how well he looked. I expected him to be almost unconscious but he was fairly alert, all things considered. His only problem was that every time he tried to get up his front legs crumbled underneath him. And he would yelp whenever I tried to flex his swollen wrists. He didn't show evidence of pain anywhere else.

"You should have seen it," began his owner, Todd Cash, a big, young athletic guy with a crew cut.

"He was chasin' this one pigeon and he's such a fool he just wasn't thinking. He lunged at the bird and went sailing over the edge. It must have been thirty metres. Then he hit the deck hard. It was sickening. He was out cold. I was dead-set sure he was gone."

"He's lucky not to be," I said.

"Yeah, by the time we got around to him he was liftin' his head up a bit. That's when your vet mate told us to bring him here. He said you wouldn't mind."

I could imagine how Rob would have said that.

"I think what's best is if you leave Tyson with us now, and we'll treat him for shock and pain this evening and get some X-rays of those wrists in the morning."

We carried him into the hospital proper on a stretcher, and settled him into one of the cages. I took a moment to check on Pepe, who was showing some interest in all the commotion that was going on. That was an encouraging sign.

The next day we took some radiographs and Tyson had severely dislocated the bones in both wrists. It wasn't simply a matter of putting it all back in position and setting it in plaster. It was far too unstable for that.

We referred Tyson to the Sydney University Vet School who performed major surgery to stabilise both joints. It meant that he would have stiff wrists for the rest of his life but considering how far he'd fallen in his impersonation of Superdog, I thought he was pretty lucky.

chapter 14

Love is blind

People assume that because you're a vet you love all animals and that consequently you will love every creature that walks in the front door of your hospital. The obvious analogy would be that every doctor would love every patient (in the platonic sense of course) that walked into his or her surgery. I'm sure there are some patients that doctors can't stand. Similarly, while I love animals generally and my profession as a whole, there are certain animals that I occasionally see that inspire very little affection from me.

Judy Butler-Smythe sat quietly erect in her seat in the waiting room with a shoebox on her lap. Holes had been punctured into the cardboard sides and lid. Obviously a budgie, I thought, although I couldn't hear any fluttering.

She was thin lanky girl, probably in her mid twenties, with an unusually long neck and what I considered a strangely small head. Her features were angular although not necessarily unattractive, a long thin nose shadowing thin lips and a pointy chin. Her attire was very much low-income punk. Her hair was long and dark, at least it was on one side of her head. On the other side it was short, spiky and orange. Her make-up was what I am told is called Gothic — tragically pale skin with dark, almost black lipstick. She wore laddered black tights and a short green-and-white striped skirt. Her feet were bare and must have been cold, since it was early winter. To complete the ensemble she wore a baggy purple sweater. She looked like an emu in drag.

To top it all off she had earrings in abundance, although that term is a misnomer here as they weren't restricted to her ears. There were about half a dozen up the side of each ear, but two also in the side of one nostril and one in the centre of her lower lip. And if you thought that was the last of her adornments you only had to wait until she spoke to see the silver stud she had implanted in her tongue. My first thought was how difficult it would be to kiss someone carrying that much hardware.

"Come in, Miss Butler-Smythe," I said, thinking how decidedly unButler-Smythe she looked.

As she walked past me I was still waiting to hear the fluttering in the shoebox. It didn't come.

"Your bird doesn't seem to be making much noise. He must be quite sick," I said.

"It's not a bird. It's me rat, Cedric," she said, with

what sounded like a broad Cockney accent.

"'E's got this big lump on 'is 'ead and 'e's not eaten much the last few days."

Now I've never understood why anyone would want a rat for a pet. I would have thought that since the Bubonic Plague wiped out fifty million people in Asia and Europe in the 1300s the popularity of rats would have waned a bit. You'd think people would shy away from a little four-legged creature that could commit genocide. However, I'm told by some of my rat-owner clients that they make great little companions even though you can't take them for a walk around the block or for a trip out to the country in the back of your ute like you can with a dog. They won't playfully chase seagulls on the beach either, unless they're dead. And when I've asked if they sit on your lap while you're reading or watching television, I've always got no for an answer.

"Then what do they do?" I ask. "Do they just playfully spread disease?"

"They just hang out."

So does a pot plant, I'd think. And it makes less mess.

I opened the lid of the box and there was Cedric sitting quietly amongst a fair amount of rat poo. He was a black and white rat. I wondered if they called them Harlequins, like they do with black and white Great Danes.

He had a huge swelling on the right side of his face.

"OK, Cedric. Let's have a look at you."

I grabbed him firmly by the head and shoulders, remembering the very first time I ever had anything professionally to do with a rat, during my stint as a locum in Wales.

A man had brought in his two pet rats and proceeded to lull me into a false sense of security by telling me not to worry because neither of them bit. He had hardly finished speaking when one of them immediately latched tightly onto the tip of my right index finger and wouldn't let go. No matter how hard I tried to pull him off me he just would not let go. Much to the horror of the owner, who watched his rodent hit the deck, all I could do was fling him violently with a sharp downward thrust of my arm. Thankfully the rat was unhurt.

The fact that it was "most unusual for him to do that" did little to relieve thc pain in my finger or the fear that I would now probably die from any one of a dozen exotic diseases. I rushed off to the doctor for a tetanus shot.

"What about leprosy, gangrene, cholera, gout, typhoid or some other weird and wonderful plague-like disease? Don't I need a shot for those?" I pleaded.

He assured me that none of that was necessary, but I'm certain that experience had a lasting effect on how I now view all rats, including Cedric.

So I'm holding Miss Butler-Smythe's rat and looking at his inflamed swelling, his horrible long yellow front teeth becoming evident as I examine his face.

"Be careful with him," Miss Butler-Smythe said

anxiously. "He's me favourite little man."

"That swelling he's got is a very nasty abscess," I explained.

"How would he get that then?"

"I don't know. Maybe an injury of some sort. Do you have a cat?"

"Ooh no. It'd kill him."

Just a thought.

"So what can we do for him?"

"We'll have to lance it and squeeze out as much of the pus as we can. We can do it under a general anaesthetic, which could be a little risky. Or we can do it with him awake, which might hurt him for just a second."

"We'll do it with him awake if it's safer."

I walked into the surgery to grab a scalpel blade and a number of gauze swabs while Cedric's besotted girlfriend comforted him.

"It's only going to hurt for a second but it's for your own good," she whispered into his ear as she kissed him. And not just a quick peck either. The lip contact was unquestionably protracted. As she did it all I could think about were those big yellow front teeth.

I asked Miss Butler-Smythe to hold her Cedric firmly while I quickly lanced the abscess. As soon as I had, a quantity of foul yellow-green stuff oozed out.

"I love you. I love you. Yes I do, you brave little soldier," she kept saying, kissing him all the while.

Her lips were getting perilously close to the site of the infection. I wasn't sure what was making me sicker, the abscess or her unsanitary display of affection. What if the ring on her lip accidentally touched the putrid yellow-green stuff? The thought was untenable.

"Be careful not to get too close," I implored.

"It's all right. I won't catch nothing off him."

I'd warned her. What more could I say. If she dropped dead in the next few hours from some overwhelming rat disease it wouldn't be my fault.

After a few minutes I'd massaged as much of the infection out as I could.

"We'll give him a shot of penicillin now," I explained. "That should last about three days, so I want you to bring him back then because he'll probably need a second shot and we can check on how it all looks then too."

Judy Butler-Smythe was back in three days as instructed. She was wearing a pair of laddered navy tights, a red skirt and a black sweater. Her toenails this time were also black. I didn't remember seeing that fashion statement on the first visit.

Cedric was dressed the same as before. Black and white fur, yellow teeth and bald pinkish-white tail. But his face was back to normal size now.

I gave him his last injection and couldn't squeeze anything more from the abscess site.

"He's back to his old handsome self again isn't he?" she said happily.

If ever the adage "Beauty is in the eye of the beholder" was appropriate, this was certainly it.

chapter 15

Death wish

Over the years working as a vet I've come in contact with many aggressive animals, both cats and dogs. Cuddle Pie, for instance (who appears elsewhere in this book), was a vicious individual by any standards. Then there was the maniacal Kitty Imber, a ferocious feline who could not be examined outside his cat basket. His owners simply described his symptoms, a towel was then thrown over him and what was considered an appropriate injection was given through the towel. Yet in all my years in practice no animal has ever come so close to absolute evil as Digger Jones. If rabies existed in this country, you'd swear he had it.

Digger was not what you'd really call a pet, at least not according to my definition. He was a demented, battle-scarred Bull Terrier, a bloodthirsty incarnation of the devil. His owners were the Joneses, an elderly couple whose relationship with him was, to say the least, questionable.

He was so totally homicidal that even his owners couldn't get anywhere near him. In my experience most vicious animals are aggressive only toward people they don't know, and otherwise docile and loving within their own family unit. Digger Jones was a dangerous exception. He was as menacing and ferocious with his permanently wary owners as he was with outsiders. For this reason he was kept in a sealed concrete yard at the back of their home. The Joneses had a 1.5-metre high fence built to separate this area from the rest of the backyard. Digger's food was passed under this fence at meal time and the dish not retrieved until he was sleeping in some other area of the yard.

I'd been out to see Digger on a number of occasions, but fortunately, or perhaps obviously, had never had to perform any sort of detailed examination on him. It would have been an impossibility anyway.

His problems were primarily itchy skin ailments which could be assessed reasonably well from a safe distance. Treatment for this was cortisone, and if necessary, antibiotics in his food. Washing him was obviously not an option, although from time to time he was hosed down at a distance. Even at these times he would frantically attack the water jet.

Digger also suffered recurrent conjunctivitis, which was treated by Mr Jones squirting a mixture of saline and eye ointment through the fence into his face in the hope that some of it would land in his eyes.

The simple truth was that Mr and Mrs Jones were absolutely petrified of Digger. They never patted him, never took him for walks or had any loving physical contact with him at all. From my vantage point I really couldn't see that he gave them any joy whatsoever, unless of course one regards the adrenaline rush of a "near death" experience as joy, and at Mr and Mrs Jones's age that seemed unlikely. The relationship between a human and a dog can, and should, be one of the most rewarding and enjoyable experiences we can have. But this one was a nightmare, an absolute disaster of monumental proportions.

Mr Jones once recounted an occasion when, as Digger slept, he had ventured quietly into the lion's den to sweep some leaves. On waking and seeing him, Digger had backed him into a corner and bailed him up for half an hour snarling and growling. He was only able to escape when his captor became bored and finally walked away.

During one visit, following one of my volcanic, long-distance examinations of Digger that left us all shaking and palpitating, I suggested to Mr and Mrs Jones what I thought would be a welcome alternative to their lives of constant terror.

"Have you ever considered having Digger put to sleep?" I asked. "Either of you could get seriously hurt. It really might be kinder for everyone concerned."

Their reaction was startling.

"Oh no, we couldn't do that. We love him too much."

I reeled back on my heels. What was there to love? I looked across the fence at this frothing, snarling, malevolent creature and could see nothing remotely lovable. I looked at Mr and Mrs Jones still shaking in their boots from our last encounter. Our ideas on love and affection were obviously very different and I never broached the matter again.

One Friday evening Mrs Jones rang about a problem Digger was having with his ears.

"When would you be able to come over and have a look at Digger's ears?" she asked. "He's scratching them and shaking his head all the time. He's been doing it for a few weeks now."

"I'm going away for the weekend, Mrs Jones. Will Monday be all right? Or I could pop over tonight after work if he appears really distressed."

"No, Monday will be fine," she said. "He's had it for a while anyway, and it doesn't actually seem to be getting any worse."

My life had been pretty good up until then. By and large I hadn't had too many regrets, but I definitely regretted having arranged this house call. What was I thinking? How was I possibly going to examine his ears?

I arrived at the hospital at 8.30 on Monday morning with the unenviable task of telling Eliza we had to go out and look at Digger's ears. I knew she wasn't going to be overjoyed with the idea. She'd been out with me on one of my other visits there and couldn't understand why I'd even bother with such an animal.

"Eliza," I started nonchalantly. "We have to go out on a call today. I'll probably need an extra pair of hands."

"Where, and what time?" she answered, as she cleaned some of the cages. "I have a grooming booked in for today."

"It's just out to the Joneses' house," I said, as innocently as I could. "I have to take a look at their dog's ears."

For some cowardly reason I avoided mentioning the crucial point, the very reason I needed an extra pair of hands to simply look at a dog's ears. The Joneses could have been anyone, and Eliza didn't immediately relate their name to any dog in particular. It was stupid really. She was going to find out soon enough who I was talking about.

"Why do you need me?" she asked. "Do we have to get a blood sample as well or something?"

"No, it's just that the dog can be a bit of a handful sometimes," I mumbled as I walked away.

Eliza hadn't been out to the Joneses' house for well over a year. Maybe she had forgotten the level of viciousness we would be dealing with here, I thought. Then something must have clicked.

"This is Digger, isn't it?" she said bluntly to the back of my head as I kept walking.

"Yes." I braced myself for the explosion.

"You're kidding! How do you figure on doing that? You know what he's like."

I was now in defence mode.

"I told Mrs Jones to pick up a dozen sedatives on the weekend. That's enough to knock down a hundred-kilo dog, and Digger's only about thirty."

Eliza wasn't buying it and, despite the fact that I'd prescribed more than triple the dose, I really wasn't confident either. We weren't dealing with a normal life-form here.

"Yeah, we'll see," she said with a damning leer. "Have you got accident insurance? Death cover?"

Having thus rallied my troops around me I was ready to spring into action.

The call was scheduled for about two that afternoon. I had instructed Mrs Jones to give Digger all the sedatives at once, in food, about an hour or so before I was to arrive. The plan was that with him heavily sedated I could give him an injection of an even stronger sedative to knock him out completely. I realised that the sedative tablets had only been partially successful with that other horror, Cuddle Pie, but Cuddle Pie was double the size and had been given less than half as much as I'd prescribed for Digger. I felt we had a reasonable shot at it.

On the drive over Eliza said nothing. She just sat there looking straight ahead, clenching her jaw. I tried to break the silence.

"Do you reckon this will work?" I asked.

"No."

It wasn't much of a drive after that. Her silence wasn't encouraging. We arrived at the little brick cottage and knocked at the door. Mrs Jones let us in.

As we followed her down the dark hallway, she said: "You know those tablets I got for him the other day? Well, they haven't done anything to him. Had no effect at all."

Eliza tapped me on the shoulder from behind. "Good career move, Tone," she whispered.

We arrived at the backyard, where Mr Jones was waiting for us. Digger was waiting there too. He didn't look as bad as I'd imagined, so I figured the sedatives must have had some effect. I slowly walked closer to the fence. His fence. His domain. He stared at me unblinking and his lips started to curl and the growl grew from the depths of his bowel. I could see his heart pounding against his chest. I could feel mine. As I got right up to the fence he suddenly lunged at me with his entire arsenal. The furious snapping, the rabid frothing from the mouth, the demented barking. It was the whole catastrophe. I jumped back instinctively and took a moment to regather.

I looked across at Eliza for support. I got none. She had her arms folded and was looking at the ground in disgust. She didn't say anything. She didn't have to. Her face said it all. "I told you so, you fool."

The dilemma now was how to get close enough to give Digger the more powerful sedative injection.

Looking across at him I could see he must have bitten his tongue during his frenzied attack. The saliva streaming from his mouth was now bloodstained, his look even more satanic. This was someone's pet, the object of their love? It was unimaginable. It was ludicrous.

"We're going to have to lasso him, Eliza," I said, trying to control my bladder. "I think that's the only way we're going to do it."

"Your call," she said, her arms still folded.

Despite her less than enthusiastic manner at this point, I knew that when push came to shove I really couldn't have better help. She had little fear of most animals, although Digger would certainly test that, and was exceptional when it came to helping with animal restraint. Her disgust was not so much about what we had to do, but that we should have to do something at all. Like me she couldn't see that this monster served any useful purpose or had any redeeming features at all.

"Do you have a rope, Mr Jones?" I asked. "I think that's the only way this is going to work."

While he looked around in the house I prepared the injection. Double the usual dose. There were risks with that, I knew, but the risk to the rest of us if the sedative was not completely effective was even greater.

A few minutes later Mr Jones returned with a long, rusty chain. "I couldn't find a rope, but I think this will probably be stronger anyway."

The troops again gathered for their briefing. The plan was to throw the looped chain around Digger's neck and pull tight quickly. Then wrench the chain over the fence for extra leverage so his head would be held firmly against it and he couldn't turn and bite anyone.

I handed Eliza the syringe and with the chain in hand I again approached the fence. Predictably, Digger flew at me with a violent rush and I threw the noose. It hit him harmlessly in the head and landed next to him on the ground.

"Good shot."

I didn't have to turn around to know who'd said that.

I pulled the chain back but not before Digger had tried to tear it away from me. I tried several more times with little success. Soon fear and trepidation became replaced by anger and frustration. I kept making the loop larger, and finally on the sixth or seventh try I managed to get it around his neck. I pulled the noose tight quickly and dragged the chain over the fence.

"Quick, Eliza. Drop the needle and grab this and hold it as tight as you can."

As expected she was fantastic, on her knees and pulling with everything she had.

"Can you give her a hand, Mr Jones?"

Digger was throwing himself around like a hooked marlin, his head pulled tightly up against the fence. The noose was so tight our catch was starting to turn blue. If we held him too long like this he could conceivably suffocate and die. For just a second that seemed a tantalising option. I quickly picked up the syringe and jumped into his yard with it and grabbed his back leg. I gave him the injection and jumped back out. My chest was about to explode.

"OK, guys, let go now," I screamed.

The skin on Eliza's hands was torn and bleeding in places but she said nothing. In the thirteen years we've been working together I've never heard her complain.

We all watched as Digger doggedly fought the effects of the sedative. He would drop down and then get up again. He did this several times, but finally he was asleep. I ventured over the fence and approached my quarry carefully. He was out cold.

As I looked at his ears and saw that both were badly infected, it occurred to me that all this effort was probably to no avail. It was going to be impossible for anyone to put ointment in his ears twice a day for a week. So I flushed them out as thoroughly as I could and completely filled them up with ointment. I also gave the Joneses antibiotics to add to his food. I hoped it would all be enough.

As we left Digger looked so peaceful. I wondered if I'd overdosed him. I almost hoped I had.

It would be four years since Eliza and I had cheated death looking at those ears before we were to see Digger again. Mrs Jones had been in to the hospital several times in the interim to pick up his "scratching tablets" and the drops for his eyes, but we'd not made any further home visits, the last being more than enough for anyone's lifetime.

"Tony. It's Mrs Jones on the phone," Eliza said. "You remember? Digger's mum. And she's crying."

My first thought was that he'd finally caught old Mr Jones and killed him. I had macabre visions of Digger contentedly chewing on the poor bloke's dismembered arm in his concrete domain.

"Hello, Mrs Jones. What's up?" I asked.

"It's Digger. I think he's dead. He's just lying on his side not moving at all," she sobbed into the phone. "Could you come over and have a look, just to make sure."

"Is he breathing?"

"I don't think so."

I don't think so? It wasn't a trick question.

"Is his chest going up and down?"

"No. But could you come over just to see why he died," she pleaded in some distress.

"Of course I can. I'll be over this afternoon."

I couldn't understand why she was so upset. They'd as good as been living with Sadaam Hussein for over a decade. You'd think they'd be thrilled about getting half their yard back. Finally, sweeping up leaves wouldn't constitute a death wish.

"Is he dead?" Eliza asked hopefully.

"Sounds like it."

"Yes!" she said, pumping her fist as though she'd

just won set point at Wimbledon. And then realising that that was probably an inappropriate gesture in response to someone's grief she gave an embarrassed grin and walked off.

A few moments later she returned with a quizzical look on her face. "What does she want you to do?"

"She wants me to go out, assure them that he is dead and if so tell them what he died of."

A little later that afternoon I grabbed my house-call bag and started out.

"Be careful!" Eliza yelled out as I was leaving. "It might be a trick. He's not like other dogs."

I arrived at the Jones's house and was greeted at the door by a tearful Mr Jones, his eyes moist, red and swollen. He lifted his glasses and with an already moist handkerchief wiped away his tears.

"The missus is out the back with Digger," he said almost inaudibly. "She's taken it pretty badly." I followed him down the poorly lit hallway. "It's knocked me about a bit too, I've got to admit. I'm going to miss him."

Miss what? The daily walk around the block? They never did that. The trip in the car? I suppose that'd work if you hired an armoured van. Cuddling up on the sofa together watching television? After ten seconds of that there'd only be one of them left holding the remote control. The "welcome home" joyful lick on the face? The only lick you'd ever get from Digger was if you tasted any good.

We continued out into the backyard. There was

Mrs Jones standing next to a very dead Digger who they'd placed on the garden table. When she looked up and saw me she burst into uncontrollable tears. Mr Jones then gently put his arm around her quivering shoulder and began to cry again too.

While I felt for their sorrow I just couldn't understand the basis for it. It was like mourning the ending of a hurricane. Oh Lord! Please lash our coastline, buffet and destroy our homes and threaten the lives of our loved ones for just a bit longer!

It didn't make sense. Finally they could put away the medication for their blood pressure, and they were miserable. They were inconsolable because the very essence of evil was finally at rest. I'm sure if I'd searched diligently I would have found three sixes tattooed somewhere on Digger's body.

"Do you think someone did this to him?" Mrs Jones asked, having regathered herself a little.

While anyone who'd ever seen Digger might be a reasonable candidate for committing such an act, I didn't think it was likely. He was old now and, judging by what looked like an abdomen full of fluid, I thought it was either heart failure or some type of abdominal tumour.

"Can you do an autopsy?" Mr Jones asked.

Another unusual request, considering Digger's age. You wouldn't ask for an autopsy of your grandmother if she'd died peacefully in her sleep at the age of ninety-six.

"If that's what you want," I said, "but I think it's

either heart failure or cancer of some sort."

"We'd just like to know," Mrs Jones quietly added.

So I picked Digger up, carried him to the car and drove back to the hospital.

The autopsy confirmed heart failure, and so Mr and Mrs Jones could now rest easily knowing there had been no foul play. For the first time in some thirteen years they could expect to have stable blood sugar levels.

chapter 16

Performance art

John and Margaret Trapp lived in a warehouse and had a couple of Bischon dogs, Beethoven and Josephine. They spoke often of wanting to have a litter of puppies from them.

John was an artist of apparently quite some note, both on canvas and in the area called performance art. Performance art is a mystery to me. It seems to mean someone dressing up strangely or painting themselves and then doing odd things like sticking sharp objects into various body parts while snotty people walk by and intellectualise the exhibition more than it perhaps warrants.

I remember going to the opening of an exhibition of photography by the very famous Robert Mapplethorpe. At the entrance were three nude models, two female and one male, painted from top to toe in white paint and their bodies and limbs wrapped around each other. The two young women had gold rings in sensitive places, places where one would generally be unlikely to find gold rings. Every so often the performers would alter their positions and then maintain that pose like statues for some time longer.

I asked Rob and Annie, who had invited me to this show, what these three were doing. They explained it was called performance art. So much for that, I thought. I wondered if, like other artwork, you could buy it, take it home, and hang it on your wall. Imagine that. A work of art you had to feed three times a day — and be sensitive to its mood swings.

John Trapp was fairly tall, probably in his forties, and usually wore baggy clothes on his largish frame. But his most obvious physical characteristic was that he only had one arm. In one of his more notorious shows he pretends to have two and then proceeds to cut the fake one off much to the horror of his shocked audience as fake blood spurts everywhere. Performance art is an acquired taste.

His wife Margaret was, I imagine, about the same age. She looked small next to John, although in reality was probably of average size. She had an attractive, somewhat crooked smile and a generally happy disposition. I don't know what she did professionally, but I do know that she was very proud and supportive of John's work.

I'd been to their second-storey warehouse on a number of occasions and often quizzed John about some of his paintings. Many appeared very dark and morose, which surprised me because he seemed such a happy, normal guy, his public amputations notwithstanding. Others of his works were so large you had to wonder who would ever have a house large enough to hang them. These, he explained, were for galleries rather than private homes.

The time came for Beethoven and Josephine to become acquainted in the biblical sense and so fulfil the dreams of John and Margaret, who had no children of their own.

"Do you think she'll have any trouble giving birth? Do you think she'll be a good mother? Will it change her personality? Will she get her cute figure back?"

And the most common question of all prospective parents: "Do you think we're doing the right thing?"

Unfortunately I couldn't give Margaret a decent answer to any of these concerns, except that a personal trainer might help with the figure.

"All I can say," I reassured Margaret, "is that I've never had to do a Caesarean on a Bischon and as far as I know none who have had pups have had any dramatic changes in their personalities."

I didn't feel, in her anxious state, that it was wise to mention one particular Bischon mother that had bitten the heads off her pups at birth. I was certain it was merely an isolated case and not a breed characteristic.

So, all parties having been reassured that it was the

right thing to do, we set off together on the road to parenthood.

The first stumbling block was one we hadn't even considered. Beethoven and Josephine had over the years become too familiar and, unlike their clucky parents, didn't see their relationship in that way. They saw themselves essentially as just flatmates and good friends and didn't think it wise to take their alliance to a sexual level. They were obviously aware how sex changes things and didn't want to jeopardise what they had.

Margaret phoned the hospital.

"Tony, it's hopeless. When she's half in the mood he doesn't want to know about it, and when he's even a little bit excited she just snaps at him."

"Isn't that always the way with married couples."

"So what am I going to do?" she asked plaintively, not responding to my weak attempt at humour.

"You and John don't stand around watching, do you?"

"We just want to make sure nothing goes wrong."

"What could possibly go wrong, Margaret? Dogs have been doing it for centuries without you up till now. Give them some privacy. Maybe they're shy. But I do have one other suggestion. Perhaps you should take that huge dismal painting down from the wall. That would turn me off sex forever."

"Oh, Tony. John loves that one."

But I had convinced her that the two lovebirds should be left alone, with mum and dad just peeking from behind the door every so often to see if they would eventually do what comes naturally. But in a few days there was another phone call.

"It's no good, Tony. She doesn't like him."

Margaret sounded so tired and disappointed. I wondered if she'd been up all night peeking. I tried to console her.

"She likes him, Margaret. She just doesn't love him."

That went right over her head too.

"And anyway, Tony, I think she's coming off heat now. So we've probably missed the boat this time."

"You're probably right. It's been nearly two weeks. Maybe it'll work better next time. You know, different chemistry and all that stuff."

"I don't know if I want to go through all this again. It's so frustrating and disappointing."

"Come on, Margaret. In half a year you'll be chomping at the bit to have another go. You know you will."

Six months or so later Josephine was on heat again and this time strutting her stuff like a hooker. Beethoven was very much more interested and excited too, his behaviour bordering on a felony.

"Should we do anything differently with them this time?" Margaret asked, as if somehow it had been her fault that their previous romantic evenings had fallen flat.

"Besides giving Josephine stilettos, a garter belt,

black stockings and an X-rated video, I think we pretty much covered our bases before," I said.

"Tony, I'm serious."

"No, don't do anything new. Beethoven's obviously into it. Give him a chance to work his charm."

Of course Beethoven had no charm whatever. This time around he was behaving like a first-time adolescent — all saliva and misdirection. He'd probably even forgotten Josephine's name. And what did he care, anyway. When it was all over, he wasn't going to want to talk to her.

"OK. We'll leave them alone," Margaret agreed. "Josephine certainly seems a lot more receptive than previously."

A couple of days later Margaret rang again.

"They did it! They did it!" came the excited shriek over the phone.

"Is that you, Margaret?"

"Yes! It was fantastic! Beethoven was wonderful. I mean for his first time and all. He missed a few times. But we've all done that, haven't we?"

I suppose we all had, but I'm not sure it's something you'd admit publicly.

"And Josephine was so accommodating. Just stuck her tail up like a Kings Cross callgirl and stood there. Must have thought 'if you can't lick 'em, join 'em', so to speak," she added with a giggle.

"And did they tie?" I asked.

"You mean did they stick together? Oh yes, for about ten minutes. What a funny system that is.

What if one of them wanted a cigarette?" Margaret's relief was palpable as she giggled again.

"Well, that's the first stage over," I said. "Let them go at it for another few days to increase the chances of Josephine getting pregnant. I'm sure Beethoven won't mind."

"Not unless he has a heart attack, the little maniac," said Margaret. "Now, after they've mated over the next few days, what do I watch for?"

"A glow in her cheeks and a contented serenity in her eyes."

"No, really. Do I have to look for anything special?"

"Just make sure she's eating well, and let me have a look at her in four or five weeks so we can make sure she's pregnant."

"You mean after all that she still mightn't be? My God, I couldn't go through all that a third time."

Margaret's enthusiasm suddenly deflated like the air out of a balloon.

"It's possible," I said. "But let's be positive. If she starts craving ice-cream and Epsom salts, you're home free."

"OK, I'll be positive. She is pregnant, she is pregnant."

About five weeks later Margaret and Josephine came to the hospital. Josephine was looking a little tubbier than I remembered.

"She's got a bit of a tummy hasn't she, Tony?"

Margaret said confidently. "And look at her rosy cheeks."

I examined her on the table and, apart from her enlarged abdomen, her breasts were bigger too. I palpated a little deeper and could feel definite enlargements in her uterus.

"Yes, she's pregnant," I proclaimed.

"I knew it. I just knew it. And look at her eyes. The contentment of a born-again Christian."

"Now here's the deal, Margaret. The pregnancy is fifty-eight to sixty-three days, but usually toward the latter. If there are any problems at all, you have to let me know. I don't care when."

"What sort of problems?"

"Problems getting the puppies out," I answered. "If she's in labour and straining with no result for two hours or more, call me. It means she may be having some difficulty."

"I'm sure everything will be fine. Won't it?"

I'm a big one for gut feelings, and mine were swirling around like a monsoon.

I had a feeling the seas ahead weren't going to be calm, and that three to four weeks from now Josephine and I were going to be spending some very intimate time together.

"Tony. It's Margaret Trapp on the phone," Eliza called out from the waiting room.

It was around 6.30 pm. I looked at the calendar. Yes. It had been about nine weeks since her dogs had made out like Burt Lancaster and Deborah Kerr on the beach.

This phone call could only mean I wasn't going to be watching any TV tonight.

"Hi, Margaret. What's up?"

"It's Josephine."

Why didn't that surprise me?

"She's had two pups, but I think she's having trouble with the next one."

"What's she doing?"

"Well, she's straining just like with the other two, but nothing seems to be coming out."

"Are you sure she's got any puppies left?" I asked.

"I think so. Do you think you could come around and have a look?"

"Sure. We're just closing up. I'll be around shortly."

I collected what I thought I might need in my house-call bag and jumped in the car, the thought of an impending Caesarean never far away. I arrived at their home and knocked at the street-level front door of the large grey warehouse. John came down and opened up for me.

"G'day, Tony. How are you?"

Shaking hands with John was not the simple subconscious response a handshake usually is. You had to be careful to offer the right one.

"I'm well. How's our little girl?"

"Not too happy. She's resting a bit better now. But she still hasn't produced anything. Margaret'll be able to fill you in a bit better upstairs."

I followed John up a steep flight of stairs and into the open kitchen-cum-living area. Josephine was lying in her cordoned-off maternity ward, two little pups snuggled in close to her. Beethoven had worn a path into the floor with his constant pacing.

"She's really tired now," said Margaret. "But she was straining for ages before you got here."

"OK then, let's have a look at her."

I put on an examination glove with a little lubricating gel and stepped over the small enclosure wall that Margaret had set up around Josephine. I began my examination to see if I could feel a pup when Beethoven came over and put his head over the edge to check what I was doing. If I moved he'd move so as to get an unobstructed view.

"Get out of it, Beethoven!" yelled John.

Beethoven looked up at him. "What's the matter?" his bewildered expression seemed to say.

"It's OK," I said, as I gave him a little pat on the head. "He's not bothering me."

Beethoven looked back at John. "See, I knew I was allowed to be here," he intimated by his arrogant pout. Then he put his head over the edge again and resumed his job as medical ombudsman.

I continued my examination. There was another pup with its head just in front of the pelvic inlet. It was the last one. I couldn't feel any others further up.

"How long has she been resting?" I asked.

"She stopped straining just after I spoke to you on the phone," Margaret answered. "So I suppose it's been about half an hour or so. Is she going to be OK?"

"Well, you were right. There's another pup in there."

I took off my glove and squatted on my haunches.

"I'll first give her a shot of Oxytocin," I told the three worried parents. "That will help her to contract more forcefully and maybe get that pup out without any further intervention. I'd like to avoid a Caesarean because the pup is so close. It'll be effective for about twenty minutes."

I gave Josephine the injection. Now it was just wait and see.

"So, John, have you done any more paintings lately?" I asked, hoping to break the tension.

"Yes, a few. Do you want to see them?"

"Sure, so long as they're not going to plunge me into depression for a week."

He laughed and took me over to a picture of a mutilated face.

"What's that?" I asked, knowing full well his explanation would have nothing to do with what I was looking at.

"It's a self-portrait."

"Of you?" I said mystified. "When? After a head-on collision?"

John laughed again. He was probably used to the reactions of cultural philistines like me. He then showed me another picture consisting of random splashes of colour, mostly in dark, sombre tones.

"And that one?" I asked.

"Self-portrait."

"Of course. How stupid of me."

A little further along the wall he pointed out another canvas on which a bunch of squares were painted, some overlapping, others isolated.

"Don't tell me. Self-portrait, right?"

"Yes," said John. "I'm doing a self-portrait study at the moment."

"That's ridiculous. You could do anything and call it a self-portrait. Isn't it supposed to look like you, at least marginally in some way? I mean, shouldn't it at least look like a human?"

"It's all a matter of interpretation."

I looked at my watch. I'd been attending to my cultural growth now for about twenty minutes so it was time to have another look at Josephine. Putting on another glove I again felt inside her and now I could feel a little head starting to pop through into the vagina. The Oxytocin had been of some benefit.

I looked around at Beethoven, who had his head over the edge again and was staring intently with a furrowed brow. This was always a difficult period for first-time fathers.

"What do you think we should do now, doctor?" I asked him.

He just wagged his tail for a second and then went back to being concerned.

"So what do you think, Tony?" Margaret asked.

"Well, she's pushed it a little further. I'm going to

try and gently pull it out the rest of the way."

I handed her the other two pups. "Would you hold onto those for a minute?"

She took them from me and held them up to her breast. "They're so small and beautiful," she purred, staring blankly ahead like da Vinci's Madonna.

Back to the matter at hand I managed to get a couple of fingers around the pup's head and very gently applied a little traction. You have to be very careful not to pull too hard. I once had a phone call from a woman who'd tried to do it on her own and pulled on the head with a little too much zeal. Well, anyway . . .

As I pulled, Josephine groaned and contracted more forcefully. This was difficult for her.

I gave her a rest so she could catch her breath. Margaret was breathing more frequently and forcefully too, especially when exhaling. The Lamaze technique she had practised at Josephine's antenatal classes was now obviously proving of benefit.

"How long between your contractions now, Margaret?" I asked flippantly.

She just looked at me a little embarrassed.

John was standing next to the fridge trying to appear composed, but sweat on a cold day is always a bit of a giveaway.

"So, how's it going, Tony?" he asked quietly, with just a hint of total panic starting to surface.

At this point Margaret couldn't say anything because she was going into oxygen debt.

"Margaret. It's all right," I said reassuringly. "We'll get this little one out."

I placed my fingers into Josephine again and this time managed to get them around the pup's shoulders. Applying gentle pressure, and with the help of Josephine's renewed contractions, I pulled slowly and cautiously. The pup was gradually coming through. I placed my fingers further down its body and pulled again. We did this pull and relax a number of times until finally the pup popped out. A healthy little girl.

"Give the man a cigar," I said, holding his daughter up to Beethoven.

He just sniffed the pup and looked perplexed. He didn't know quite what to do now that the ordeal was over. He was probably too caught up in the excitement of it all.

I gave the pup back to Josephine, who immediately began licking and cleaning her. The little one was making puppy noises and immediately began looking for the nipple.

"Put the other two with her now, Margaret."

She was flushed as she placed them next to Josephine.

"It's wonderful, isn't it," she whispered, as all three pups began to drink.

I looked across at John, who was still trying to maintain his masculine I-was-never-worried poise, but it seemed to me that you don't grab tightly onto the fridge door if you're coping. And your knees aren't bent when you're standing.

I wondered if, despite the emotional havoc he had just survived, this introduction to the marvel of birth and fatherhood would now inspire John to move from self-portraits and create a whole new series of paintings. Not that any of them would even remotely resemble what we'd all just witnessed. Maybe if we were able to give Beethoven some paint and a brush we might get closer to the truth.

chapter 17

On another plane

"What's your name?" Eliza asked as the plump lady presented herself at the reception desk.

She was, I suppose, somewhere in her mid thirties, but she looked so strange the margin for error could have been a decade either way. Her hair was cropped short but not evenly all over. It was as though she had attacked it with a pair of scissors without going anywhere near a mirror. A sudden urge to create a new but poorly advised image. Her cheeks were flushed but not in a healthy way, and her eyes sometimes had that faraway dull stare that suggests that she spent much of her time in some other distant cosmos.

Today she wore a large black Demis Roussos-like caftan, and over her right shoulder she carried a blue Ansett travel bag, although I'm sure her travels weren't on that airline's flight paths.

"Astral," I overheard her say to Eliza.

"Is that your name or your cat's name?" Eliza asked.

"It's my name," she replied, as though it should have been obvious.

"Astral who?"

"Just Astral."

"Oh, so that's your surname."

"No. It's my only name. I decided to shed anything extraneous in my life." Like a grip on reality.

I could see the look of contempt on Eliza's face. She had little time for such alternative lifestyles. "Thank you," she said, politely but curtly. "Take a seat. Tony will be with you in a minute.

"Miss Astral?" I asked of the closely cropped black tent sitting alone.

She walked past me and into the consulting room like some famous diva, chins and nose triumphantly in the air, her blue wriggling Ansett bag still over her shoulder. She was shorter than I'd expected judging from her sitting height. As she passed I could see what an incredible mess she'd made of her hair. I couldn't believe that anyone would purposely go for such a moth-eaten look.

She placed her moving bag on the table.

"It's not Miss. Just Astral," she explained. "I don't want to burden my life with the weight of extra names or titles."

I could see the sense of that. I had three names and my life had been hell.

"So, Astral," I managed, "how can I help you?"

"It's my kitten. He's not well," she said, unzipping the bag and releasing a bright-eyed, bushy tailed three-month-old bundle of ginger fur. "I don't know exactly what's wrong with him."

I looked at the purring, playful little creature that was now mischievously pawing at my pen. I couldn't see what was wrong with him either.

"His name's Stratosphere," she said, adjusting the shoulder area of her robe that the Ansett bag had left creased.

How appropriate, I thought, to name your pet after one of your favourite holiday destinations.

"Nice name," I replied.

"I called him that because he's way out there," she said with a slight chuckle.

People in glass houses . . .

"What appears to be wrong with him?" I asked, directing my attention back to the matter at hand.

"He's not well. Look at his eyes."

I looked at his eyes. They looked wonderfully alert and sparkling. Then I began to examine the rest of him.

"Is he eating?" I asked.

"Oh yes, he eats everything."

"Is he sneezing?"

"No."

"Any diarrhoea or vomiting?"

"No."

"Is he playful or lethargic?"

"Really playful. He runs up the curtains and hides

behind doors and attacks me when I walk past."

So far this didn't sound like a kitten on the critical list.

"I'm giving up smoking," Astral then confided.

I looked up from the kitten. "Excuse me?"

"It can't be good for him, all that passive smoking. I'm going to get those patches. You know, the ones you stick all over you, so your body thinks it's having a cigarette."

I wasn't sure how many patches she intended buying, with that description.

"That's a good idea," I said. "Smoking's not too good for any of us."

I continued to look over the healthiest kitten I'd ever seen.

"I smoke for my nerves," she admitted. Then after a lengthy, somewhat agitated pause accompanied by what I perceived was the occasional twitch, she said, "But I'm much better now."

I looked across at her. Somewhere there was a psychiatrist who hadn't earned his money.

"And I don't want my cat to die of lung cancer."

I made a few mental calculations. Like how long a cat generally lives and how much cigarette smoke one person alone could generate in a house. I figured cats lived about twelve to fifteen years on average and passive-smoke-induced lung cancer was very unlikely in a teenager. So unless she spent all her waking hours blowing smoke directly into her cat's face I felt her fears, while well intended, were probably unfounded.

"Well, Astral," I said reassuringly, "I think it's great that you're giving up smoking, but I don't think you need worry about giving Stratosphere lung cancer."

"He's a Scorpio and I'm a Virgo, so I hope we get on together. Those signs aren't very compatible, and you know what Scorpios are like."

Now, I'm a Scorpio and I didn't think I was all that terrible. But we were talking about a cat here, and I wasn't sure how astrological considerations really came into it.

"I'm sure you two will get on just fine," I said.

"Does he need antibiotics?"

"Antibiotics?" I asked, bewildered. "What for?"

"You know, to make him better."

Better than what? Stratosphere was now in orbit half way up my stethoscope. He was using the metal part of it as a chin-up bar.

"Astral," I said, starting to get in the swing of that name. "There's nothing wrong with him. He's well. He's a healthy, happy little kitten. All he needs is his first vaccination and worming."

"Yes, I think he's given me worms."

I decided to give that one a wide berth. I knew he couldn't have. And besides, it was nearly lunchtime and to ask her to describe her symptoms would mean I wouldn't be able to eat until dinner at the earliest.

"Well, it's just as well we worm him then," I said, hoping to defuse a potentially unpleasant situation, and proceeded to give Stratosphere his injection and his first dose of worming.

"Maybe he needs some pain killers," Astral suggested. "Don't you think he looks a bit sore?"

Stratosphere demonstrated his obvious pain by jumping onto my shoulder from a standing start.

"No, Astral. A vaccination and worming are all he needs right now. Nothing else. No antibiotics, no chemotherapy, no dialysis, no heart transplant, no nothing. You've got yourself a robust, bouncing little kitten. All we have to do is see him again in a month for his second vaccination."

"Or before that, if he gets sick again," she said earnestly.

Krug was the friendliest, largest, handsomest Bull Terrier I'd ever seen, although handsomeness was not a term most people would use to describe a Bully.

With their big, parrot-shaped heads — and Krug had the biggest — and tiny little beady eyes, they certainly were an acquired taste. And with the exception of Digger Jones — who was Charley Manson perfected — they were generally the most gentle creatures with people. It is only with cats and other dogs that they could sometimes become less sociable, if homicide can be considered antisocial.

Krug had, for some time, suffered a sore shoulder and this made him bear weight unevenly on the corresponding foot. This in turn had led to the formation of painful corns, and this was the main reason he would visit the hospital. We'd removed them surgically but that only provided temporary relief as they would soon recur due to the chronic shoulder problem. Finally, anti-inflammatory softening creams appeared the best method of controlling his symptoms.

He came in fairly regularly for vaccinations and check-ups for his feet, and it was always a joy to see him. He'd rock into the consulting room like a happy Rumanian weightlifter. He was bow-legged only because his muscles were so big, and his joy at seeing me was completely unbridled. This was a dog seemingly incapable of creating mayhem.

Robyn McCrea, his owner, was a tall athletic blonde lady who'd once landed badly from a parachute jump, smashed her ankle and ended up in plaster for God knows how many months. To watch them both hobble into the surgery was the stuff of silent movies.

Once in the consulting room she would let Krug off his lead so he and I could commence our man-to-man greeting thing. I'd grab his huge head in my hands and put it close to mine and pull away just in time as he tried to lick me. We were like a couple of Masons at the start of one of their brotherhood meetings. He loved the whole repetitive procedure. His tail would accelerate to a blur. After a few minutes of such male bonding we'd get down to the serious job of examining each other.

The consulting room and waiting room are connected by a two-way swinging door. I figured it was the best design to allow people easily through, while at the same time dividing the two rooms. The folly of that design was soon to become evident.

It was just another one of Krug's regular visits, this time for his yearly vaccination. We'd finished with the formalities of our blokey welcome and I was walking over to the fridge to get his vaccine, when I heard the front door of the hospital open. Krug also heard it. What I didn't know then, but was soon to discover, was that a slender young lady had walked in with her joyful, not-a-care-in-the-world, little Cavalier King Charles Spaniel prancing by her side.

Krug suddenly got a strange glazed look in his eyes and stood peculiarly mesmerised by the swinging door. His tail had stopped wagging as he focused forward, unblinking. I'd never seen him like this before. You could have hit him over the head with a four-by-two and he wouldn't have blinked.

Then something in him snapped and he was off, straight through the swinging door using his head as a battering ram. The sound when he hit it was like the explosions that made the French unpopular. He didn't slow down at all to negotiate it. Just straight through.

Robyn screamed, "Krug! Stop!"

But how do you stop a torpedo? How do you tell Joe Louis "Don't hit him!" when the left hook is half way there?

Krug was on his way. Once past the door he sped towards the reception desk where Eliza was sitting, bolted between her legs, nearly knocking her off her chair, and attacked the Cavalier like a marauding Viking.

All I could hear was shrieking and yelping from the owner and her dog.

"Tony! Quick!" Eliza yelled.

I ran out to find Krug attached to the smaller dog's ear and shaking his head violently. The slender lady was trying to pull her dog away.

"Pull him off!" she kept screaming. "Get him off!"

And the spaniel kept snapping. Frantically, everywhere, trying to free himself.

I tried desperately to open Krug's jaws but it was impossible. His grip was far too tight. I just wasn't strong enough. I knew I shouldn't have had a haircut the day before.

Robyn hobbled in next. "Krug! Let go! Let go!" she shrieked as she also tried to pull him off.

But he was well and truly beyond that. He had the single-minded focus of a religious fundamentalist.

There was blood everywhere, and I was afraid that if we couldn't stop this mayhem we'd soon be left with an ex-Cavalier.

Amid all the screaming and snapping, Robyn miraculously had the idea of grabbing Krug's testicles. Apparently this was a common tactic, the Bullies opening their mouths either in ecstasy or agony depending on the pressure applied. Whichever it was wasn't important, just so long as the final result was achieved.

Once Robyn had grabbed firmly, Krug instantly

let go. He looked around, startled, I assume in order to work out who to thank.

Immediately we pulled him away and the slender lady pulled her little spaniel away too.

Robyn dragged Krug back into the consulting room while I stayed in the waiting room to see what damage he'd done to his little victim. I was so sure it was going to be horrendous, what with all the blood and everything. But surprisingly, there was almost nothing. Krug had spent the whole melee solidly attached only to the ear of his prey and hadn't managed to damage anything else. Even that ear was only bruised and swollen. There were no cuts or abrasions. So that made me wonder where all the blood had come from.

I looked at the slender lady whose face was now as white as a ghost. Eliza stood there with a comforting arm around her.

"Are you OK?" she asked, rubbing the woman's shoulder.

"Yes, I think so," she said.

But she wasn't. In order to be OK your complexion should be a bit rosier than the White Cliffs of Dover.

There was blood streaming from puncture wounds on both her trembling hands, all inflicted by the frantic, random biting of her own dog as she tried to rescue him. She was obviously going to buy her heart-worm tablets elsewhere in future, perhaps in a demilitarised zone.

"Come upstairs," I offered. "We'd better get those wounds cleaned up."

"Thank you. But I don't think they're all that bad," she said feebly. Her hands continued to quiver.

Tin Legs Bader had probably said something similar after his plane crashed.

"All the same, it's better we have a look," I insisted.

I washed her hands gently in disinfectant. There were about half a dozen punctures and a lot of bruising. They looked so sore. She couldn't stop them shaking. Her face had become even paler, if that was possible. The last time I'd seen anyone that pale, people were throwing flowers on him.

"I want you to go straight to the doctor up the road and get those wounds looked at properly," I instructed. "And then you must let us reimburse you for your medical costs."

I figured that was the least I could do, having left her anaemic from an over-the-counter sale.

Having seen her out of the hospital and directed her to casualty I went to have a look at Robyn, who was back sitting with Krug in the consulting room. He was acting like nothing had happened, wagging his tail and wanting to swap stupid handshakes again. He'd had a great time, even if everyone else looked like they'd just stood on a landmine. But I wasn't in the mood. He was in my bad books for the moment.

Robyn was bleeding from her hands too. Not as badly as the other woman, but badly enough.

"Do you have any penicillin allergies?" I asked.

"No. Why?"

"Because you're going to need some antibiotics. You can either go to the doctor or you can take some of these. They're the ones I take if I get bitten," I said, taking some tablets off the shelf. She was a client of long standing and so I felt it was all right to offer.

"How is she?" Robyn asked of the Cavalier's mum as I cleaned her wounds.

"She's OK," I said. "I've sent her up to casualty." A contradiction if ever I'd spoken one.

"And her dog? Is he all right?"

"Yes. He's only got a sore ear. Pretty lucky really."

"Oh dear," she said. "I'm so sorry. It's just not like him. I don't know what possessed him."

"It's all right, Robyn," I reassured her. "It's not your fault. These things happen."

But of course these things shouldn't happen.

"I'm going to have to get a latch fitted to that door in the future," I added.

So, having tended her wounds and ignored Krug's unwanted attempts at reconciliation (he was far too happy and smug with himself), I saw the two of them out of the surgery, and slumped back into my chair. I was physically and emotionally drained. I felt like a cigarette except I didn't smoke. I felt like a drink except I didn't drink.

Eliza walked in with a cup of tea. "Here," she said. "You looked buggered."

So I sat looking at the ceiling with the cup in my hand. I kept thinking how much worse it could have been. I was so glad it was all over and I could relax again. The worst of the day was over. I half nodded off.

"Tony," Eliza called out. "It's Astral on the phone. She says her cat's sick again."

It's times like these you start to question the existence of a compassionate God. You begin to add up the good and the bad deeds of your life and wonder if the balance is favourably tilted.

I picked up the phone lethargically. "Hello, Astral. What's up?"

"He's sick again. The same as the last time."

"Astral, he wasn't sick the last time."

"But he is this time. He looks really funny to me. I think he's having an emotional crisis," she said anxiously. "Can I please bring him down?"

I'd just survived the afternoon with Pol Pot, and now they were sending me one of Sigmund Freud's case studies.

"Of course you can, Astral. Come straight down."

It had been three months since Astral had last been in (she'd forgotten to get Stratosphere's second needle even though we'd sent her a reminder). She walked in just as operatic as before and sat down with the same old blue Ansett bag. She adjusted the haircomb in what was now becoming a more luxurious growth. The caftan today was floral, which went nicely with the ug boots.

"Hi, Astral," I said, with the resignation of someone who knows what is about to befall him but is powerless to prevent it. "Let's have a look at Stratosphere."

"He's not called Stratosphere any more."

"Of course he isn't."

"I decided to change his name to Baby because that way I'd feel more like he was my child."

"You don't think that's putting too much pressure on you?"

"Oh no. I love children."

My instincts had been correct. This was not what I needed so soon after escaping the trenches of Tobruk.

"So what's wrong with Stratos . . . I mean Baby?"

"He seems, well, sort of, you know, not well."

"In what way not well?"

"You know. Not himself."

I looked at the now older kitten who'd escaped from the bag. He looked as tragically ill as the last time. He was purring as he brushed affectionately against me.

As I bent down to commence what was obviously a pointless examination he rubbed his face on mine.

At this point Eliza walked into the consulting room to get something off the shelf. "He doesn't look well, does he, Astral?" she said, sneaking a wink at me.

"No," Astral replied earnestly. "He doesn't."

"So what specifically is the problem, Astral?" I continued, ignoring Eliza.

"Well, I have to move out of the house soon and I think he senses something."

"Is he eating? Is he still playful? Does he appear to be in any pain?"

"Not exactly. He just seems concerned."

How concerned can a six-month-old kitten be?

"And anyway," she went on, "I'd like someone with a farm to look after him for two years while I look for a new house. Do you know anyone?"

"Do I know someone with a farm to look after Baby for two years?" I repeated.

I wanted to be absolutely sure what I'd heard. And why specifically two years?

"But I'd want visiting rights. You know, legally."

Oh dear. A custody battle.

"I'm sure a magistrate would look at your position favourably," I said.

"When I was in the music industry I knew five-hundred people. Had them all on computer. Anyway, I got out of that business."

What? Did I miss something? I could no longer keep pace with her. I continued with Baby, who, as expected, was perfectly healthy.

"I could have asked any of them to look after Baby," she continued, "but you see more people than I do now, so I thought you'd know someone."

"Look, Astral," I said, sidestepping the surrogacy issue. "I really don't think he's too sick, but he does need his second vaccination so why don't we give that to him now."

"OK, but do you think I should take some medicine home with me just in case?"

"What type of medicine would you like?"

"Just something that makes him better when he's sick."

I began to wonder if there was such a thing as Feline Munchhausen's Syndrome by proxy.

I vaccinated Baby and delivered a bit of a lecture on why it wasn't a good idea to give medicine willy-nilly.

Astral never did move out of her house and Baby came in a few times each year, purred, caressed and dribbled with delight — all the signs of a cat that had, unfortunately, only fifteen years to live.

chapter 18

Blind faith

Martina and I sat down to our takeaway lunch of pasta and tomato soup from the little Italian restaurant up the road. This had become a bit of a Thursday ritual for us, provided the workload for the day allowed us the time. Martina had just pre-meded the surgery cases in the hospital and that gave us forty minutes or so to savour our banquet.

So there we sat, in the surgery office, scooping up lashings of *penne melanzane* with huge wads of Italian bread and listening to the radio station that plays all the old favourites that I love and Martina has never heard of. Just as we had settled in for the long lunch, the idyllic moment was shattered by the harsh noise of the phone ringing.

I looked at Martina. She looked at me with a mouthful of pasta and a stupid grin.

I was at a disadvantage. My mouth was empty.

I reluctantly got up from the table and answered it.

"Hello, it's Tony Sheldon here. Can I help you?"

"It's Monica Soo. My father just phoned me and said his budgie was very sick."

"What did he say the problem was?"

As I said this I glanced across at Martina to make sure she wasn't eating more than her fair share. She looked up only to get a breath between mouthfuls and caught sight of me watching her. She smiled wickedly, took an unnecessarily large scoop of pasta and slowly, almost sensually, put it in her mouth. She closed her eyes in mock ecstasy. I was going to have to deal with this phone call quickly or starve.

"He says it's not singing any more," Monica continued. "Would you be able to go out and have a look at it for him today?"

"That should be fine," I said, still being tortured by Martina. "Is your father home all afternoon?"

"Yes, he never goes out much any more. He's quite old." Then there was a pause. "By the way, his name is Charlie. The budgie's name, that is."

I quickly wrote down the address, assured Monica that I would be around that afternoon, and then hung up the phone and rushed over to the table and confiscated what was left of lunch. Martina had made a sizeable hole in it.

"You've had your half, you little glutton," I said.

"What do you mean? There's much more than half left."

But her smirk betrayed her honesty and I ate

standing up so that this piranha couldn't ravage what was left.

When I'd eaten what I considered my fair share I sat down and we continued as we'd started out — sharing amicably.

"What have we still to do this afternoon?" I asked.

Martina looked at the daybook. "We've got to stitch up Fatty Grant, and we have to X-ray Luther Stanton and maybe put his leg in plaster."

Fatty Grant was an aptly named obese Basset Hound who had cut his leg pretty badly on something in the park. He was the pet of Roger Grant, a distinguished young gentleman who always wore a coat and tie irrespective of the weather. Roger explained to us that Fatty had two great passions in life — eating and scent-following. Obedience was toward the bottom of his list of priorities, if in fact it was on the list at all.

Fatty had, apparently, been on one of his single-minded scent sessions in the park when Roger noticed blood on Fatty's hind leg. He managed to get close enough to notice it was a nasty gash, about ten centimetres long.

"Silly fool didn't even know he was cut," Roger chuckled. "Just kept on sniffing. Of course he didn't come when I called him for a closer look. He's never done that in his life. Why should he start now?"

Roger had somehow been able to grab Fatty, who wasn't that fast due to his massive girth and short legs, and carry him back to his car. He had the sense to bandage Fatty's leg with some cloth to control the bleeding before he brought him in to us.

The wound was deep and, after all the mud and grass Fatty had been through, wasn't too clean either. It took quite some time to clean all the muck out of it and then stitch him up with several layers of sutures. We then bandaged the leg with a fluoro pink bandage. We figured the very conservative Roger Grant would like that.

Luther Stanton on the other hand was a cheeky six-month-old cat, a Devon Rex who looked like ET. He had very little hair on his body and almost none on his head. He'd fallen two floors while swiping at butterflies from the balcony of his apartment. He didn't seem overly perturbed by his accident, except that he couldn't use his left back leg. He continued to rub his bald little head affectionately against anyone who came within striking distance, and never stopped purring. It felt to me like he'd broken his tibia. X-rays confirmed a fairly nasty break and so Luther was sentenced to four weeks clomping around the house with his leg in plaster.

I was fairly confident of Luther's recovery, having been enlightened by a lecturer at a Salt Lake City veterinary conference of a syndrome known in the United States as New York Disease, which refers to the habit cats in that city have of regularly falling out of the windows of high-rise apartment buildings. Fortunately, we were told, cats' bones heal very quickly, much faster than dogs'; and we were assured by the lecturer that, as long as we managed to get all the broken pieces somewhere in the same room, the limb should heal. Of course, he said, that was providing the cat wasn't dead, in which case the healing would be slower.

We had Luther in for weekly cast check-ups and he'd quickly adapted to his new peg, walking and running effectively by swinging the big white club around in wide arcs to compensate for his being unable to bend it.

By the time I'd finished with these two cases it was about two o'clock. Plenty of time to go and visit Mr Soo and his budgie.

I drove around to the apartment block and knocked on his ground-floor door. There was no answer. I waited a considerable time before knocking again, this time more loudly.

Soon the door opened and there stood Mr Soo, a tiny little Chinese man. He must have been in his mid seventies, his hair thinning and silver. He was dressed in a white short-sleeved shirt and dark blue baggy pinstriped trousers with braces. He wore leather sandals with white socks. And he carried a white cane. A long white cane. It was a just a minor point, but one I felt his daughter perhaps could have mentioned, if only in passing, to fully prepare me for the visit.

"Hello, Mr Soo. I'm the vet."

He bowed his head in Eastern acknowledgment. "Ah good. Come in. Please. I am happy you here."

As he looked up I saw the opacity of his eyes, just like the teacher in Kung Fu. They looked straight through me, and yet there was a gentle serenity about him, a calm which seems unique to ancient Eastern philosophy.

"Very good you can come. Bird very ill. Not say anything last few days." As he said this he pointed his cane to the bird cage. "Charlie over there."

I walked over as Mr Soo sat down in a large chair, holding his cane between his legs.

I looked in the cage.

Charlie was on his back with his feet in the air. It was obvious he had lost more than just his voice.

"You help Charlie?" Mr Soo asked plaintively.

I took Charlie out of the cage. He was as stiff as a board. He looked like he had been dead for days. I couldn't understand how Mr Soo could have missed it, even if he was blind. Surely he would have noticed Charlie wasn't eating or flapping his wings or jumping around. Perhaps he just didn't have any actual physical contact with Charlie and thought that he was just very quiet because he was ill.

It then occurred to me that he'd have no idea what Charlie looked like.

"Charlie's very sick," I said.

The die was now cast. Having lied I could no longer turn back.

"You think he die?"

"I don't know, Mr Soo. I'll take him back with me to the hospital and see what I can do."

I stuck little rock-hard Charlie in my shirt pocket and headed out. "I'll call you if anything happens."

"Thank you, thank you," Mr Soo said, bowing his head frequently.

I rushed straight to the pet store and asked the shopkeeper if she had any male budgies who were good talkers.

"What colour would you like?"

"It doesn't really matter," I said. Under the circumstances that seemed a pretty safe bet. But I pulled Charlie out of my pocket anyway and showed her. He was green and yellow.

"I've only got a blue male at the moment," she said. "Do you want to wait until we get a green one in?"

"No, a blue one will be fine."

I took him back to the hospital in a shoebox and transferred him to a proper cage.

"Is that Mr Soo's budgie?" Martina asked.

"No, his is dead. This is the replacement."

"Did he ask you to get him a new one?"

"No. He doesn't know his is dead. I took his bird away and said we'd try and make him better. If this one talks OK, I'll take him back to Mr Soo and tell him Charlie's cured."

"Sure," Martina said sarcastically. "And he won't notice the difference. What, is he blind or something?"

"As a bat."

"You'll get caught. He'll know somehow."

Ignoring Martina's scepticism I placed Charlie II

and his cage in the kennel room and waited and hoped.

We kept him for a few days to make certain he was a good talker. Sure enough, this little budgie was a veritable raconteur.

Satisfied that the bird could pull off the scam I drove back to Mr Soo, having phoned him earlier with the good news that I'd managed to bring Charlie back to good health.

He'd been elated.

"Thank you. I thought I lose him," he'd said. "You make me very happy."

He'd been so overjoyed I was starting to feel the first pangs of doubt. What if he could tell the difference? How would I explain it? This had to work. I was in too deep.

Mr Soo greeted me at the door, bowing continually. "I'm so happy, so happy. Charlie a very good friend."

"He's much better now," I said convincingly. "We nearly lost him." Now I was making myself sick.

I carefully took the new bird from the shoebox and put him into the cage, where he immediately began jumping from perch to perch as though he had always lived there. Charlie II started eating his seed with relish.

Mr Soo walked over and joined me at the cage. This was the test. I held my breath.

"He sound much better. He very happy again." Mr Soo held his ear close to the cage and smiled.

The benevolent deception had worked. I could breathe easily again.

"You must call me straight away if he gets sick again, " I said as I opened the door to let myself out. "We may not be able to save him next time if you leave him so long again."

"Yes. Thank you, thank you. Very happy now." He bowed a few hundred more times as I left.

I arrived back at the hospital, content that I'd done the right thing.

"So, did you get away with it?" Martina asked.

"Worked like a charm. He didn't suspect a thing."

A few days later Martina called me to the phone. "It's Monica Soo. She wants to talk to you."

Martina was a little too smug for my liking. I wondered what could possibly have gone wrong. Surely Charlie II wasn't sick or worse. It had only been a couple of days. I took the phone with some trepidation.

"Hello, Monica. What's up?"

"Hello, Mr Sheldon. I just rang to thank you for fixing up Charlie. My father's so happy he's better."

"Oh good, I'm so pleased," I said with some relief. "Charlie was pretty sick."

The thing about having started a lie is you have to be very careful not to deviate from the storyline.

"Yes, he sure was. I was over at Dad's place yesterday and he says that whatever medicine you gave Charlie made him talk more than ever."

"Isn't that fantastic," I said.

"And, Mr Sheldon, that medicine must have somehow changed the colour of his feathers as well." Her delight at my expense was unmistakable.

Of course, how stupid of me. She would have seen Charlie many times before.

"Oh dear," I said. "The fatal flaw."

She was laughing on the other end. "It's OK. It was a nice touch."

chapter 19

Over the fence

We all have those days when, for no particular reason, we're depressed. The weather is good, home life is good, business is good . . . but there's no spark. It's like you're walking around with your head in a dark cloud.

Whenever I found myself drowning in one of those days of self-indulgent misery, I would hope for a Mrs Moss house call. It's not that she had such fantastic pets. Far from it. She had an old flea-ridden, skinny black Labrador-cross and an equally skinny old black and white desexed tomcat. She, herself, was a little brick of a lady. Mid sixties with poorly dyed, short, curly jet black hair. Not more than 150 centimetres tall and almost as wide. She had thin tight lips and wore bright red lipstick well outside the margins to make them look fuller. She had no eyebrows except for the ones she had drawn in. Her little city terrace was always immaculate, which surprised me as her animals were always filthy.

But Mrs Dorothy Moss was off with the fairies. A real nutter, but not your standard crazy. She appeared, on first impression, quite normal in almost every aspect. Her speech was normal. There were no involuntary head movements, or sudden glances at imaginary flying objects. She did, I suppose, seem unusually wary, but I put that down to the neighbourhood she lived in. It's just that she would say things that would suggest that her grip on reality was at best tenuous. And it was these journeys into uncharted territory that took my mind off my own woes.

My first contact with Mrs Moss really should have tipped me off.

Eliza was working in the cattery that day, so I answered the phone.

"Hello. It's Mrs Moss. Can you come around and have a look at my dog? He's pissing everywhere. I can't stand it."

I took a moment to digest her graphic account of the problem. Some people only have one way of describing bodily functions.

"Goodness. We'd better stop that then," I said. "What's your address?"

"What do you want that for?" she snapped back. This should have been enough to start a few alarm bells ringing.

"So I can look at your dog."

"You won't give my address to anyone else will you?"

"Of course not, Mrs Moss," I reassured her. "But it is a fairly important piece of information for a house call."

She reluctantly gave me her address, but not her phone number.

"They'll all listen in if you give them a chance," she said.

I had no idea who "they" were, but I was soon to hear much more about them.

I hung up the phone and called out to Eliza. "Have you ever spoken to a Mrs Moss before?"

"Oh yes. She rings here occasionally. Never gives us any details though. Why?"

"I have to go out and look at her dog."

"Have fun. I don't think she's the full quid."

I arrived at Mrs Moss's immaculate little terrace, and was shown through to the kitchen where her old dog, Bill, had settled on a blanket in the corner. He looked up at me, gave a couple of lazy thumps with his tail and settled back.

"What are they poisoning him with?" Mrs Moss asked somewhat angrily.

"Why do you think he's being poisoned?"

There didn't appear to be any symptoms to suggest that. As far as I could see, all Mrs Moss had was an old dog with a bad case of flea eczema, who for some reason wasn't controlling his bladder too well.

"Because he never did that before. They're poisoning him. I know it. That's why he's pissing everywhere."

"Who are 'they'?" I asked, cringing a little.

"All those foreign people who've moved into this area. They put all this black stuff into the air and over my fence," she explained in disgust.

This was definitely starting to approach weird. I glanced out her kitchen window and saw no evidence of the "black stuff". No sign of it on her pavement either.

"I don't see any black stuff," I said, peering into the never-never.

I soon learnt not to question Mrs Moss's theories. But this was my first visit and I didn't then know that she was often inclined to imagine things.

"The black stuff was there yesterday," she said. "And they'll throw more over tomorrow. They wouldn't do it if my husband was still alive. And they're not doing it now because they know you're here."

"Well let's hope they stop it soon," I said sternly.

That effectively ended any more discussion about "the foreign people" and the mysterious "black stuff", and I settled into examining Bill. Apparently he would dribble urine as he walked. It wasn't that he was consciously urinating in the wrong places or more frequently than usual. He just dribbled.

His problem turned out to be an enlarged prostate, and due to his age and generally poor condition we opted for hormonal therapy instead of castration to reduce its size, at least until we could get him in better physical condition. We could do surgery later.

The treatment worked well and the problem had settled within a few days, although I don't think Mrs Moss ever really accepted my medical explanation. As I explained the problem to her she would just say "Yes, yes" and continue to look suspiciously out the window.

Over the years Mrs Moss's stories became stranger and stranger and pretty soon I found myself shamefully looking forward to those visits, wondering where I would be taken on her next flight of fancy. It was sad, though, that all her imaginings were paranoid. She was convinced that someone was always trying to hurt her or her pets in some way.

On another occasion I'd arrived to look at her cat, Tom, who, she complained, had terrible breath. Upon looking in Tom's mouth the reason was obvious. He had disgusting teeth with a putrid plaque build-up on them. I opened his mouth to show her.

"Can you see here?" I began. "All that crusty yellow stuff on his teeth is plaque. The only way to effectively get rid of it is with an ultrasonic tooth scaler, so we'll need to have him in the hospital for the day."

She seemed to understand what I was saying, or at least said she did, and was happy for me to take Tom. I thought that was that and headed for the door with Tom in his basket. Then her demons returned.

"The teeth only got bad when they started throwing those cane toads over the fence," she yelled from down the hallway, pursing her lips and squinting accusingly. "Right where he sleeps outside by the kitchen door. He eats them and then his teeth go bad."

Cane toads over the fence? And apparently in quite some numbers, which was unusual because they are rarely found outside the tropics. Sydney, being temperate, was an unlikely breeding ground.

"Why do they do it?" she asked plaintively.

"Why do they throw cane toads over the fence? Mrs Moss, I really don't know. Are you sure that's what's happening?"

I'd just broken the cardinal rule. Don't ask questions. Don't query anything. Just listen and absorb.

"They think I don't see them doing it," she said. "But I do, and more than once too. It's not right. It's just not right."

She often ended her accusations with that judgment.

Another seemingly routine visit had veered dramatically off course. I felt it best to simply agree that no, it wasn't right that someone should throw cane toads over the fence, and bid a hasty retreat to the hospital, where I could get to work on Tom's dental problem.

"Is that Mrs Moss's cat?" asked Eliza as I walked into the surgery. "What's up with him?"

"He's been eating cane toads. Someone's been throwing them over her fence. Hundreds of them."

"Did you see any?"

"No, not one."

"Fair enough," said Eliza and went back about her business.

Tom's teeth were extremely bad and many had to be extracted. I suspected that he may also have had some early kidney trouble because he'd started drinking more water than usual. A few simple tests confirmed that his kidneys were starting to pack it in. Mrs Moss, of course, would have a different explanation for his altered drinking habits. Foolishly I attempted to explain it to her.

"Tom is starting to show signs of kidney failure," I began.

"Of course he is, with all the things they're doing to him. I tell you, it's not right."

That was my cue to suspend any further clarification of his condition, suffice to say that over time it would gradually get worse. I had a busy day lined up and as much as I would have liked to hear her diagnosis there really wasn't time. I did try to give some dietary advice that might slow the progress of Tom's complaint but I'm sure it fell on deaf ears.

It had been well over a year since my last visit and I was again called to see Tom, who'd become very thin and frail. His kidneys had clearly deteriorated since I'd last seen him. He was drinking much more water than before and I could see that we were nearing the end of the road. His face, once round and full, was now thin and gaunt due to his dramatic weight loss.

I bent down and looked at the poor bedraggled cat on the sofa. "Tom's not looking too good, is he?"

Mrs Moss slowly shook her head in anger and tightened her lips. Her lipstick was a lot wider of the margins than usual.

"He was OK until they changed his head."

That one really stunned me, which was surprising because it had been a long time since her stories had been able to do that.

"Changed his head?" I asked, eagerly awaiting some explanation.

"Yeah. Put that little skinny one on and took his nice big round one away. He was OK until they did that."

"Why would they do that?" I asked.

"I don't know. They shouldn't do it, should they? It's just not right."

So, it seemed "they" were at it again. And I suppose she was right. It wasn't fair that they should have taken Tom's nice round head away. I didn't even bother to question her theories. I simply told her that Tom, for whatever reason, was in severe kidney failure and that I needed to do some tests to determine if we'd be able to do anything to help him.

"Of course his kidneys are buggered. It's all them poisons they're throwing into my place. Green stuff. It's making me sick too."

Well, whether it was the "green stuff", the "black stuff", the cane toads or whatever, Tom was plainly beyond help and the tests confirmed it. We put him to sleep and, for a while at least, left Mrs Moss to struggle with her demons alone.

I wondered what ailment Bill would have next to take me back into her nether world.

chapter 20

Dotty about Dottie

I loved Dottie Abblett. She was one of my all-time favourites. She brought such joy to everyone she ever met. Not an unhappy bone in her whole body. And Dottie and I were to go through hell and high water together. I think that's what brought us so close.

I first met her when she was eight weeks old and coming in for her first vaccinations. It was the day after my disastrous foray into big-game hunting at Digger Jones's place. I was still suffering the effects, when in bounded a baby Harlequin Great Dane, the black and white designer type. It was Dottie, all boundless joy and unco-ordination. At that age Great Danes haven't got the walking thing figured out yet. Their feet are several sizes too big and their legs far too long for their bodies. The whole walking exercise is one of continually trying to unravel the knots their legs often find themselves in.

She bounded in, totally out of control, both physically and emotionally, frantically trying to greet every animal and person in the waiting room simultaneously. Her dog lead was of no use at all, as it was far too long to prevent her reaching anything she wanted to reach. She jumped up at the front desk, missed, and landed flat on her face. It didn't faze her one bit.

She headed straight for a grumpy old Cattle Dog who wanted nothing to do with her antics. He had an anal problem and was having trouble sitting properly. The last thing he needed was some uncontrollable tongue trying to get acquainted. He snapped at her. That made her blink in astonishment for about a second and then launch into a playful barking attack at the old codger. Dottie could never fathom the notion of anyone, dog, cat or person, not loving her and wanting to play.

"Dottie, come here. You're going to get bitten," Gloria Abblett half-reprimanded as she tugged on the lead to pull Dottie away.

Gloria was a good-natured lady in her early thirties. She was on the slightly cuddly side with thick wavy red hair, and those incredibly rosy cheeks you only see on Vegemite commercials. She smiled and laughed often, and had an unmistakable gentle kindness about her. Dottie had done well. They seemed ideally suited to each other.

Dottie's first examination was a total waste of time. When I managed to get close enough to examine her,

I was close enough to get licked or jumped on. The stethoscope was only there to be chewed. I assumed she was healthy and administered her first vaccination — a needle I'm sure she had no idea she'd been given, so taken was she by the excitement of her new surroundings. It didn't slow her hyperactivity at all. She left the hospital as effervescently as she had arrived.

Four weeks later it was time for her next vaccine. She wasn't any different, just a much larger version of the original. Still the ungainly lope, still the overwhelming joy of new company and the same sound of the ever-wagging tail hitting everything, only now it was louder.

It was wonderful how pleased she was to see me again, but then she was probably just as pleased to see anyone. Dottie wasn't overly discerning.

The vaccination and general examination went much the same way as the first. Another total waste of time, only now the tongue was larger, faster and considerably wetter. The needle again went in unnoticed and as usual she turned the entire consultation into a social occasion. I looked forward to her coming back in one month for the last of her initial set of vaccinations.

Unfortunately I was to see Dottie under much less favourable circumstances two weeks later.

It was a Sunday afternoon and I was on call. My pager went off and I dialled the number it flashed up. On the other end was a lady in a panic.

"Hello, Mr Sheldon. I'm so glad I got you. Dottie's had a terrible accident."

"What happened?" I asked, thinking how it always seems to happen to the wrong dogs.

"She's been hit by a car, and it was all my fault. I let her off the lead just as we arrived at the park and she saw another dog over the road and ran back after him. I should have waited till we were well into the park. I feel terrible."

"It's no one's fault," I reassured her. "Bring her to the hospital straight away."

Some twenty minutes later Dottie arrived.

She wasn't a pretty sight, multiple abrasions all over her body. She could walk all right, so there didn't appear to be any broken bones, but her breathing was very laboured. She was struggling, almost gasping for breath, and yet, through it all, the silly thing still made feeble attempts to wag her tail, still tried vainly to jump up and greet me.

"Get down, you little fool," I said as I gently pushed her away and tried to settle her.

Her breathing worried me, and I thought it best to tell Gloria my fears straight out.

"Dottie may have torn her diaphragm. I think that's why she's having so much trouble breathing."

"So what do we do?"

"We're going to have to take X-rays to confirm it but if it is torn then it's a risky surgical procedure to repair it."

"Oh dear, oh dear." She paused and bent down to

pat Dottie, who almost involuntarily slurped her with a somewhat slower tongue. "Well, there's not much choice then. I suppose we'd better do it."

I looked at Gloria, who had tears streaming down her face. Then I looked at Dottie looking up at Gloria. All I could think of was that this whole thing had better work out.

"OK, Gloria, leave Dottie with me and I'll call you this evening as soon as whatever has to be done is done."

She left, having given her little friend one last huge hug, and there I was left with Dottie and what felt like the weight of the world on my shoulders.

The problem now was that I needed a second pair of hands. I couldn't get in touch with any of the nurses and so I was left with my usual option in these cases — my dad. On various occasions he'd helped me with surgical procedures when no one else was available, and had done a great job. Having spent his youth on a farm he was not nauseated by the sight and smell of blood, and was comfortable handling all animals. He also enjoyed the opportunity of doing something different. I only hoped that on this occasion he'd be available.

I rang. "Hello, Dad."

"Hi, Shtern. What's up?"

"Are you busy?"

"I'm just lying by the pool, but we're going out this evening for dinner. Why?"

"I need a hand at the hospital. A Great Dane pup

has just been brought in after being hit by a car and I think she's going to need an operation. Do you think you'd be able to help me?"

"Well, Shtern, I'll have to check with Mum first. How long do you think it will take?"

"I really don't know. It depends on what I find. If it turns out to be what I think it is, then it might be a few hours. What time's your dinner?"

"I think it's about sevenish. Hold on a second, I'll just make sure."

I waited a couple of minutes, desperately hoping he'd be able to come over. Dottie's breathing wasn't getting any better. If anything it was getting worse. I pulled up her lips and her gums were looking blue. That concerned me.

"Shtern?"

"Yes, Dad. Can you come?"

"I can, but I have to be back about 6.30. Do you think we'll be finished by then?"

"I think so. I'll see you in a bit."

I hung up the phone and prepared everything for the X-rays. I decided to also prepare everything I'd need for surgery in case my suspicions about Dottie's condition proved correct.

When Dad arrived about twenty minutes later we placed Dottie gently on her side on the X-ray table and took radiographs of her chest.

The results confirmed my fears. She had a severe hernia of the diaphragm and her intestines, and probably some of her liver had slipped into the chest.

That's why she was having such trouble breathing.

This isn't one of my favourite operations. The access to the diaphragm is difficult for a start and these patients stop breathing when you open up the abdomen because, with the diaphragm torn, all the normal pressure in the chest is released. That's why I needed Dad. He would breathe for Dottie by squeezing the rebreathing bag at regular intervals.

We placed her on the operating table. Dad knew how to hold up her vein so I could give her the anaesthetic, as he'd done it a dozen times before. Dottie kept trying to lick my face as I tried to place the needle in her vein. I hated that. This was such a risky operation. I was so worried about the outcome and she just continued with that "puppy" total trust thing.

Finally we had her asleep and, after attaching an intravenous drip, the operation began.

The tear was massive. The largest one I think I'd ever seen. Murphy's law — best dog, worst hernia.

And to make matters worse she had also ruptured her bladder, a complication I hadn't even considered with all my attention directed to her breathing difficulties. That would have to be fixed after I'd repaired the diaphragm.

Painstakingly, I sutured the torn edges of the diaphragm, as Dad rhythmically breathed for her. Everything was going well, when I noticed blood starting to pool alarmingly in the chest. I had no idea where it was coming from.

"Dad, can you squeeze the bag with one hand and reach over with the other and press this swab here."

He pressed the swab on the general area where the bleeding seemed to be coming from.

"Now, when I tell you, slowly reduce the pressure," I instructed. "I should be able to find the bleeder that way."

"OK, how's that?" He released the pressure too quickly and the blood started pooling again.

"Put pressure on again," I said, this time with some urgency. We got the bleeding under control again. "Now, release a little bit slower this time. And don't forget to keep breathing for her."

Dad was certainly earning his supper trying to keep the breathing regular and at the same time concentrating on the rate of pressure release on the swab. But he kept calm. He was one of the coolest people I've ever known, and in this situation that was crucial. It took a few more goes until we got the pressure release timing right and I was able to find the blood vessel in question. I stopped the bleeding and proceeded over the next hour and a half to complete the repair. With the diaphragm wholly closed, and a thorough check for any leaks made, Dottie started to breathe on her own. The most crucial part of the surgery now over I proceeded to repair the ruptured bladder. That posed few problems compared to the earlier dramas.

I finished sewing Dottie up and we put her in a cage to recover.

"Thanks, Dad. You were fantastic," I said as I closed the cage door. "Now go and have a great dinner. You're going to be late. I'll be OK from here on in."

The smile on his face was a such proud one. He wouldn't say in so many words, but he really had a great time doing stuff like this.

"Just give me a call if you need me again," he said on leaving, his chest a little larger than I'd remembered.

The next two hours were spent anxiously sitting next to Dottie's cage waiting for her to wake up. After about an hour she started to lift her head drunkenly. She looked around through hazy eyes and spotted me. Her tail managed a few feeble wags and then it, along with her head, dropped with exhaustion.

Another hour down the track and she was half sitting up. I opened the cage door and sat with her, stroking her swaying head. Dottie was going to make it. I was so relieved. She looked at the dog in the next cage and, through the steel grid, tried to lick it too. And then she started to piddle normally. I never enjoyed cleaning out a cage so much.

"Gloria, Dottie got through it all OK," I said reassuringly on the phone. "She had a ruptured bladder as well, but that's been fixed too."

"I'm so relieved. I'd really prepared myself for the worst."

"Why don't you pop in and visit her tomorrow."

"I'd love to."

The next morning Dottie's breathing was still a little laboured but much better than it was prior to surgery. She was hungry and happy, almost like new. Gloria arrived promptly at nine and their reunion was overwhelming. Tears, laughter, tongues, tails — the whole bit. It was really too much for Dottie and so the visit had to be cut short. She was wrapping her drip around her legs as she continually turned circles of delight.

We decided to keep her in hospital for a couple more days to ensure that her activity was kept to a minimum. After that her recovery was uneventful.

A week later she returned to have her stitches removed, and bounded into the crowded waiting room without a moment's hesitation. You'd think she'd have been apprehensive after all that she'd been through. But fortunately that was never Dottie Abblett's style.

chapter 21

Captured on camera

Just up the road there's an institute that does behavioural studies on monkeys. Round pegs in square holes, that sort of thing.

Harry lives up there with Theodore, Beatrice and Megan. He's a nasty, unsociable piece of work. I'm sure they toyed with the name Himmler before settling on Harry. All four of them are macaque monkeys from Malaysia, probably out here on working visas. And they've all been having such a wonderful time they're thinking of applying for refugee status on the grounds of gorilla warfare in the jungles back home. Apparently Megan was even thinking of having a baby so she could get a bigger cage, but Theodore didn't want the responsibility.

They each have their own large enclosures, but often they're put in together to socialise and have their interactions studied. Except for Harry of course.

He's kept on his own to prevent bloodshed.

On a regular basis I'm asked to check on the health of the foursome and the condition of their living quarters. Everything is always impeccable, and I do enjoy the opportunity of visiting some of my early ancestors. It's fascinating to see where we all came from and how poorly some of us have evolved, especially on Saturday nights.

Beatrice, Theodore and Megan are always happy to see me. They jump around, showing off, squealing with delight, doing somersaults and hanging from their rings and bars. Generally making monkeys of themselves.

Harry, however, is never pleased to see me. Every time I walk past him he attacks the front of his cage like Hannibal Lecter looking for something to go with his Chianti. He snarls and shrieks menacingly and generally carries on like an opposition back bencher. I'm sure the only reason they keep him is to study the evil side of nature. A Jekyll and Hyde perspective.

It was one o'clock on a quiet Friday afternoon when a panic call came from the institute.

"Tony! Theodore's just attacked Harry. There's blood everywhere!" It was Moira the secretary, and she was shrieking. "I'll put you straight onto Damien."

Damien was the young bloke responsible for the care of all the monkeys.

"Hi, Tony."

"Damien. What's happened?"

"It's that bloody Harry," he began. "He was reaching under the divider between the cages, trying to steal Theodore's food, and Theodore attacked his hand. I think he bit off one of his fingers."

This was sounding more like question time by the minute.

"And what about the rest of Harry?" I asked.

"It's just his hand, I think. Theodore couldn't reach anything else." Then there was a moment's silence and he went on. "Do you think you could come over and stitch him up? I've already managed to sedate him, and I've got all your instruments ready."

They had a reasonable operating facility there for such emergencies.

"I'll be there in a few minutes," I told Damien, and hung up the phone.

"Hey, Martina! Do you want to come with me to stitch up a monkey?"

She was putting a cat we'd just finished operating on back in its cage to recover. "What?" she yelled back.

"Do you want to go stitch up a monkey?"

She walked out of the kennel area with the broadest smile on her face. "Really? Now?"

Martina had, for so long, wanted to see the monkeys at the institute, but we'd never been able to co-ordinate our times. She'd always been busy doing something else whenever I'd made my rounds. But because of all I'd told her about them, she seemed to know them almost as well as I did.

"So who did Harry attack?" she asked. It was an obvious assumption.

"No. Theodore got Harry," I said. "Can you believe it? He grabbed his hand and apparently tore it to bits when he was trying to steal some food from his cage."

"Serves him right," Martina replied. "He's had it coming for a long time."

She was sounding like she'd had a relationship with him.

"Anyway," I interrupted, before she could continue her tirade. "We have to go straight away. Damien's already sedated him."

We left the hospital for the five-minute walk to the institute, but after about a hundred metres Martina suddenly turned around and rushed off into a chemist's. Ah, I thought, so that explains why she'd snapped so viciously at the justice of Harry's comeuppance.

But when she emerged she had a grin on her face that made the Cheshire cat look like it was in mourning. She'd bought one of those cardboard all-in-one cameras. The ones you buy for around eight bucks and the pictures are always lousy. If it isn't brilliant sunshine everything you take looks like it's midnight.

"Just for posterity," she replied breathlessly.

"I think it'll be a bit dark for a decent picture inside."

"No, it'll be OK. I'll just make sure the operating

light is right behind me and I'll get really close."

That sounded like the makings of an ideal surgical environment, but I figured as long as she didn't come in between me and Harry while I was operating we'd probably manage.

Moira met us at the door, still in a bit of a tizz. "Thanks for coming so quickly. Damien's down the hall. Second door on your left."

"Hi, Damien," I said as I walked in. "This is Martina. She's come along to help."

Damien was sitting next to Harry, who was lying doped to the eyeballs on the operating table. He'd try to lift his head occasionally but it was all too much and he'd invariably lapse back into semi-consciousness.

"Did you have much trouble sedating him?" I asked.

"Not really. Once we finally managed to get the net over him properly and pull it tight we didn't have too much difficulty giving him the jab."

With Harry I knew it wouldn't have been that easy. He would have struggled and thrashed about like a netted white pointer, and Damien didn't look like someone who'd just been out for stroll in the park. He was bleeding from some nasty scratches on his arms and I know he's not married.

Confident that Harry was adequately subdued I bent down to have a look at his mangled hand. The pinkie was gone. The index and fourth fingers were flaccid and bent, and the central long finger was pointing straight up as though someone had cut in front of him in the traffic.

"Martina, can you hold his arm out so I can get a better look at his hand?"

You could see she was ecstatic at being part of this adventure. It was the first time she'd ever been this close to wildlife, at least among the lower primates.

As she held his arm I examined the extent of the damage to the remaining fingers. The index finger didn't have too much feeling, although under heavy sedation that assessment may not have been too accurate. The central gesturing finger seemed reasonably OK and the fourth finger was much like the index. They all had ragged, uneven tears in them as did the rest of the hand. There was also a deep wound in the area preferred for most suicides.

"Should I take a picture now?" Martina asked as if I had initiated the whole photographic concept and she was only following orders.

"Yes, now is good, but be quick."

"Look at me and smile. You get in the picture too, Damien," she directed. "And Tony, hold up Harry's hand like it's waving at me."

"Should we weigh it and nail it to the wall along with the moose's head?" I asked.

Damien and I looked at each other, then we looked unblinking at Martina.

"OK, OK," she said. "You don't have to smile."

"Martina," Damien began as she placed her camera back on the bench, "can you hold Harry while I mask him down? That way Tony can start to scrub up."

Martina held the limp body of Harry in her arms like a woman cradling a child.

"Oh look, he's so cute," she gushed as she gently rocked his flaccid form back and forth.

"He's not cute, Martina. He's unconscious. It's not the same thing," I said as I continued to scrub.

"I think he likes me."

"Look at the middle finger on his bad hand, Martina. Does that look like the gesture of someone who likes you?"

"Can you take a photo of us together before we knock him out completely?" she asked, ignoring me.

"Go on, Damien," I urged. "Take one before she starts to lactate!"

Damien took the shot and then with the mask over his face Harry was sent floating to the other side.

We lay him on the table, draped him up and I started work on the badly shredded hand. The skin was torn irregularly and several exposed tendons were either partially or completely severed. I stitched the stump of what remained of the little finger and spent the next hour or so trying as best I could to piece the rest of the mess together. Martina, in between cutting the sutures for me, took about a dozen photos, none of which I figured would be any good.

"Damien. Is this injury going to muck up any of the work you have to do with Harry?" I asked, my eyes focused intently on the job.

"Only if you screw up the surgery."

That certainly had a settling effect. "I see."

"Because if you can't get full function back to the fingers he's got left, then the institute will have wasted the fifty thousand dollars they've invested in his training."

Now, I know a certain amount of pressure is good and supposedly brings out the best in us, it's just that the added burden of someone else's impending bankruptcy hovering over me like the reaper acted more like a laxative than an incentive.

"And if that happens," Damien went on, "then we're all out of a job."

I was comfortable with that.

"That wouldn't be so bad except I'm saving up for my brother's life-saving kidney transplant. I'm giving him one of mine."

At that point I looked up to see Martina had almost bitten through her bottom lip. Damien's poker face was holding out only marginally better.

"You know, you were doing OK until that kidney thing," I said.

"Too much was it?"

"Seriously, what happens if it isn't perfect?"

"Not much really. We were going to retire him shortly anyway."

The weight of mass redundancy having been lifted, I continued the reconstruction of Harry's hand more confidently.

By the time we'd finished I was fairly pleased with

the result, although it would take some weeks before we would know how successful we'd been. The biggest risk, aside from infection, was whether Harry would leave his stitches alone. Monkeys have a habit of continually pulling and chewing at sutures until they're all out and the wound reopens. I hoped it would remain painful enough for him not to be tempted.

"Can I just hold him once more before we put him away?" Martina asked.

We removed all the surgical drapes and cleaned up the hand, after which Martina gently lifted Harry off the table and took him back to his cage to recover. There was some intense bonding going on here, except that it was totally one-sided. As gentle, vulnerable and harmless as Harry looked now, on awakening he would be quite happy to tear Martina's head off.

As soon as he saw his adversary brought back, Theodore really started to strut his stuff. He puffed out his chest, screamed, ranted and walked round like John Wayne. For the moment at least he'd reclaimed the hill. Beatrice looked like she was ready to give him her phone number.

I returned to the institute weekly to check on how Harry's hand was healing. Initially it looked like all the work had been for nothing, as it showed little increase in mobility. But I suppose I was thankful he'd at least left the sutures alone. However, as time passed, movement slowly began to return to his fingers and as it did Harry's persona again reverted to the demonic.

He showed his gratitude for Martina's care and affection by screaming and throwing his food at her.

"Can you believe he did that?" she said, wiping squashed banana from her face.

"Let it go, Martina," I replied. "You'll meet other monkeys, I promise."

The status quo had returned. Theodore again sat meekly next to Megan as his chest slowly deflated and Beatrice changed her phone number.

In the meantime Martina had picked up the photos. Every one of them looked like it'd been taken in the Jenolan Caves.